BIOHACKING AND LONGEVITY

A Practical Guide to
Optimized Health

BIOHACKING AND LONGEVITY

A Practical Guide to
Optimized Health

Dr. José Roberto Melo

1st Edition
2026

EDITORA
SUARDI

1st Edition 2026

Publisher: Giselle Suardi

Responsible Editor: Editora Suardi
Layout: Editora Suardi
Preparation and Review: Editora Suardi

Cataloging-in-Publication Data

Melo Filho, José Roberto de.

Biohacking and Longevity: A Practical Guide to Optimized Health / José Roberto de Melo Filho.
Orlando, Florida: Editora Suardi - Suardi Group USA, 2026.

Print book. Paperback.

ISBN 978-1-970481-40-2

Biohacking. 2. Longevity. 3. Health optimization. 4. Preventive health. 5. Wellness. 6. Self-care.

I. Title.

EDITORA SUARDI

Instituto Suardi
Curitiba - PR - Brasil
@institutosuardi
institutosuardi@gmail.com

TABLE OF CONTENTS

DEDICATION

***I dedicate this book first and foremost to God,** the owner of gold and silver, the Beginning and the End, the Physician of physicians.*

I dedicate it to my beloved wife, who understands my absence while I work and write this book, and who admirably devotes her life to our home and our children.

Also to my parents, who taught me, through example and love, the value of effort, faith, and integrity, pillars that sustain my entire journey.

And to my mentors, professors devoted to conveying an honest vision of medicine, especially Dr. Lair Ribeiro, who was undoubtedly my greatest inspiration at the beginning of my career.

ACKNOWLEDGMENTS

I thank my beloved wife, through whom alone I came to understand what it means to be one flesh; my mother, who taught me to be kind and generous; my father, who taught me that honesty is not a virtue, but an obligation; and Master Jesus, who held my hand and guided me toward the light while I was walking lost, who sustains me and makes me feel special.

FOREWORD

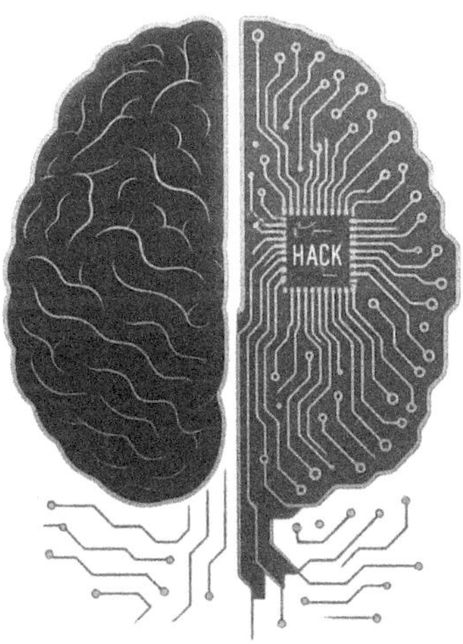

I met José Roberto Melo, to me, simply Beto, many years ago, when we shared a classroom in a postgraduate program in Nutrology in São Paulo. He was already a licensed physician, but what impressed me was the restlessness he carried within him: he did not accept easy answers or ready-made truths. He sought to understand the human being as a whole, not as isolated fragments. Since then, I have followed his path, marked by courage, study, and conviction, until he became the physician who now presents this work to the reader.

This book is the result of an already mature journey, built through years of dedication and practice. It was not born from trends, but from clinical experience combined with a passion for investigating causes rather than merely treating consequences. Beto shows that caring for health goes far beyond fighting symptoms: it is recognizing the connections between mind and body, understanding the influence of the environment, respecting the rhythms of life, and above all, remembering that medicine is not limited to prolonging days, but to giving more life to our days.

Throughout these pages, the reader will find reflections and practices on essential themes: food as a tool for health, hormonal regulation, sleep, light, movement, therapies that expand vitality, and even the spiritual dimension, which gives meaning to the journey. Each chapter is an invitation to rethink daily choices, from the plate to the routine, from discipline to rest, from technology to contact with nature, showing that longevity is not built by chance, but through conscious and consistent decisions.

What makes this work special is that it does not offer shortcuts, but paths. It does not promise magic formulas, but invites small changes that, with consistency, transform destinies. It is a book that reminds the reader that discipline is a form of freedom and that taking care of one's health is not an obsession, but a responsibility toward what we have received as a gift.

There is a passage in Job 42:5 that says, "*I had heard of You by the hearing of the ear, but now my eye sees You.*" This book offers the same invitation: to move from hearing about something to experiencing it, to transform information into practice, to let theory become life. It is allowing health to stop being merely a future expectation and become something lived in the present, in every decision.

Writing these lines is an honor. I see in Beto a physician who does not remain silent, who takes a firm stand, who upholds principles even when they are unpopular. His life, in medicine, in family, in faith, is consistency in motion. He is not intimidated by criticism, he is not led by the ease of convenience, and he does not surrender to the silence of omission. That same courage can be felt in these pages: the courage to say what needs to be said and to show that health is far more than statistics and diagnoses; it is story, purpose, integrity.

Longevity that is truly worthwhile is not merely a count of years; it is density of life. It is remaining whole, lucid, and useful, guarding the heart against the excesses that make both soul and body ill, and making discipline a quiet form of love. This is what this book insists upon, with balance: science without arrogance, tradition without nostalgia, spirituality without escape from reality, clinical care without reductionism.

To the reader, I leave a sincere invitation: walk through these pages with curiosity and courage. Question, reflect, adapt. Discover that health is not merely the absence of disease, but the presence of balance, purpose, and love. May this book inspire you to live not only longer, but better, more lucidly, more fruitfully, more gratefully. For true longevity is not stretching the calendar, but deepening meaning.

Victor Sorrentino

PRESENTATION

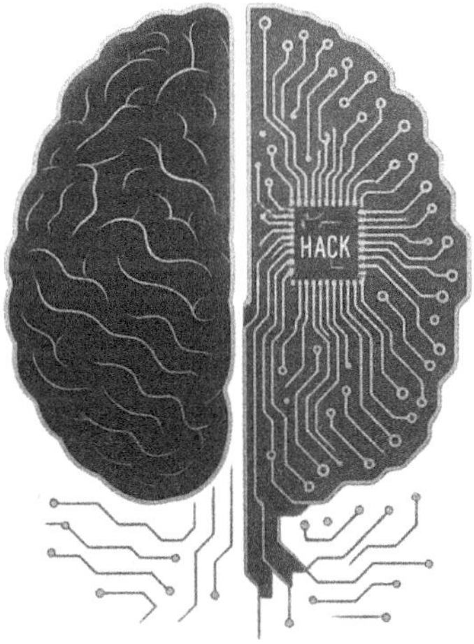

Hello, thank you for being here. I am Dr. José Roberto de Melo Filho, originally from Piumhi, a peaceful town of 35,000 inhabitants in the countryside of the state of Minas Gerais, Brazil. I am the son of Zé Beijo and Dulcy, I have three siblings, and I am married to Priscila, I have three siblings and I am married to Priscila, a virtuous woman who manages our home, our company, the Melo Institute of Integrative Medicine, and is also responsible for our children, Benjamin and Henrique, three and two years old, respectively. I also have a beautiful and loving 15-year-old daughter, Valentina, who lives far away with her mother, but is always visiting us in Belo Horizonte, the city where we live.

My journey in medicine began in 2010. Right after graduating, I moved to São Paulo. Between one hospital shift and another, living practically inside hospitals and always treating the same people with the same symptoms, I soon realized that it was like bailing out a sinking ship with a spoon. In 2012, I was a tired doctor, with only two years in the profession and no fixed routine. I still had terrible habits and sleep deprivation, and I exercised only occasionally, with no rhythm and none of the results I could have been proud of.

My diet consisted of processed foods such as pizza, quick snacks from the hospital cafeteria, fried foods, and sweets. But an angel sent from heaven, Dr. Breno Faria, a college colleague, introduced me to an introductory course for a postgraduate program. Without fully understanding it, I enrolled, struggling to pay around eight thousand reais for four days of learning focused on healthy longevity.

Those were the four most disruptive days of my life, during which the professors captured my attention so intensely that I would not have noticed whether the microphone sound was too loud or too low. I only wanted to dive deeply into that knowledge, which somehow lit a flame of hope in my heart. I was completely captivated.

After that impactful experience, I enrolled in the master's postgraduate program in Longevity Sciences. It was approximately two wonderful years that propelled me toward other postgraduate programs, such as Endocrinology, Nutrology, and Integrative Medicine, in addition to dozens of weekends spent at congresses and courses, all focused on functional and comprehensive medicine, with respect for the specificity and individuality of every human being. I studied herbal medicine, gut health and microbiota modulation, metabolomics, interpretation of laboratory tests, hormonology, and nutrition.

Faced with so many challenges, in 2014 I was finally able to stop doing hospital shifts and opened my first private practice. I no longer had to alternate between a borrowed office, where I saw patients twice a week, and the exhausting hospital shifts in São Paulo. I moved to Belo Horizonte and stayed close to my family. Even so, those first years were difficult. I remember crying in my office because I had no patients, only two or three throughout the week. But things began to change. With the results I was able to provide through humane and personalized medicine, referrals and word of mouth gave me a fully booked schedule.

My greatest professional accomplishment has been witnessing the transformation in my patients' lives throughout my journey in Integrative Functional Medicine. One of the cases that impacted me the most, and at the same time engraved in my heart that I was worthy of my parents' respect, was when my mother came to me.

That year, in February 2019, my beloved mother, Dulcy Melo, was frustrated with conventional medicine. After spending about six months with symptoms that made no sense, and after hearing a suggestion from an ophthalmologist who suspected an autoimmune disease, she sought help in Ribeirão Preto, São Paulo, from a rheumatologist. That was when she was told she had Sjögren's syndrome.

In this disease, the body's immune system attacks its own healthy cells that produce tears and saliva. She would choke, feel thirsty in the middle of the night, experience fatigue, light sensitivity, red and irritated eyes, and changes in taste, but what bothered her most was the thirst, lack of saliva, and tooth pain. My mother reported drinking six liters of water a day out of desperation because of her dry mouth.

Then one fine day, my brother brought her to my office, 250 kilometers from my hometown. When I saw her, I was shocked. Worn down, she had no voice, was weak, and was carrying a bottle of water. We spoke briefly, and I sent her to the clinic infirmary, where we immediately accessed her venous system and administered an infusion of ALA, alpha-lipoic acid, an important ally in the integrative approach to Sjögren's syndrome, especially for its antioxidant, anti-inflammatory, and mitochondrial-protective effects.

When I came across an extensive prescription and strong medications, I immediately took a stand against methotrexate and did not allow her to begin it. I also ruled out the others and followed her through the gradual tapering of prednisone, the only allopathic medication she took. My mother underwent treatment at the clinic for about 18 days. She received numerous treatments, such as von Ardenne oxygen therapy; infusions of vitamins, minerals, and antioxidants; and high doses of vitamin D. We worked with PEMF, Bemer, Biomat, Rife, ozone therapy, and others. After all this personalized care, she returned to the countryside infinitely better than when she arrived, and within four months she was in remission.

Being able to help people who arrive discouraged or facing complex conditions, such as cancer, autoimmune diseases, neurodegenerative diseases, depression, and fatigue, and seeing them regain quality of life, is something beyond measure. Today, without a doubt, the Melo Institute of Integrative Medicine is a place of healing for the body and soul. There, we enhance people's strengths, we encourage them, we modulate stress, and we closely follow every step our beloved patients climb each day.

Since founding my first clinic in 2015, I have dedicated myself to comprehensive care, treating causes and not merely symptoms. This approach has brought me regional and national recognition, but what truly fulfills me is knowing that humanized and personalized care, focused on health and well-being, directly impacts not only patients, but also their families. That certainty reaffirms my purpose and mission as a physician every single day.

INTRODUCTION

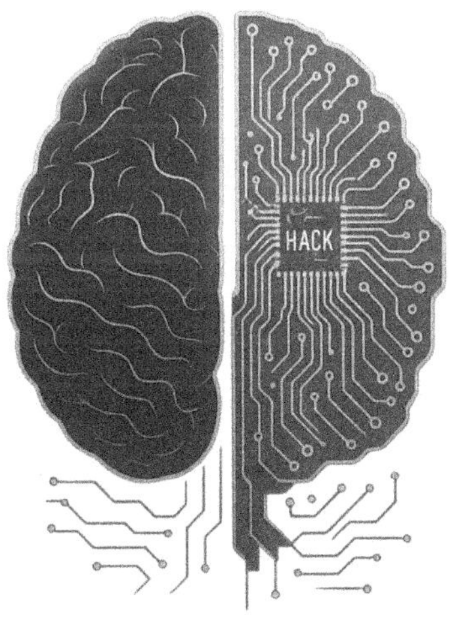

I am passionate about medicine, and for that reason I have dedicated myself to seeking solutions and strategies that contribute to the integral health of the human being. I believe in the physician-patient relationship and in personalized care, taking into account the unique conditions, needs, and circumstances of each individual in order to promote healing and mental well-being.

Conventional medicine, for decades, was built on a model that prioritizes treating disease rather than promoting health. The modern healthcare system has often drifted away from the true essence of caring for the human being and has focused on diseases, diagnoses, and medications. Instead of seeking the underlying causes of health problems, the focus turned to the temporary relief of symptoms, and patients were reduced to numbers in a bureaucratic machine, where disease became the guiding principle rather than integral health.

This model, to a great extent, was shaped by the influence of economic interests, such as the actions of powerful figures like John D. Rockefeller, who, in the early twentieth century, played a crucial role in the transformation of medicine. Through his foundation and major investments in universities and hospitals, Rockefeller helped drive the creation of a healthcare system focused on the use of synthetic drugs and on a pharmacological paradigm. In the view of some observers, this movement corrupted medicine by distancing it from holistic and alternative practices that could address the deeper causes of disease, and it turned the pharmaceutical industry into one of the most powerful controlling forces dictating the course of the world, commonly known as Big Pharma.

Over the years, modern medicine came to be dominated by large pharmaceutical corporations and a funding network that contributes to a vicious cycle. Clinical studies are often funded by these same corporations, creating a relationship of dependency that frequently distorts results. Books such as Deadly Medicines by Peter C. Gøtzsche show us the dark side of this industry, with evidence that many widely prescribed drugs are not only ineffective, but may in fact be dangerous. The indiscriminate use of medications, often without considering more natural and less invasive alternatives, has led to irreparable harm to the health of millions. We were lied to about fluoride, about Vioxx, we were lied to about OxyContin, about thalidomide, about Prozac, about thimerosal and aluminum in vaccines, we were lied to about Gardasil, we were lied to about ivermectin and hydroxychloroquine. More than 50% of negative clinical trials are not published, and conflicts of interest involving researchers are constant. This distorts medical guidelines and harms clinical decisions. A Cochrane study from 2017, "Reporting bias in clinical trials," reinforces that the data available to the public are incomplete and tend to show only the positive aspects of treatments.

This is the starting point for the biohacking revolution: an approach that challenges the traditional medical model. Biohacking, unlike conventional medicine, seeks to empower the individual to optimize health through personalized interventions grounded in scientific data. It questions the idea that aging and disease are inevitable and offers tools to increase quality of life, longevity, and mental health.

The concept of healthspan, healthy lifespan, has become a central goal, in contrast to the excessive focus on lifespan. While lifespan simply refers to the number of years lived, healthspan involves living those years with health, energy, and quality of life.

Recent studies have reevaluated the impact of traditional medications and revealed that many treatments once considered universal solutions may, in fact, be contributing to a rapid deterioration of health over the long term. The classic example of medications such as nonsteroidal anti-inflammatory drugs, NSAIDs, used to treat inflammation but known for their serious side effects on organs such as the kidneys, highlights how conventional medicine can often prioritize pharmaceutical profits at the expense of patients' well-being.

It is in this context that a new approach to health emerges: biohacking and longevity. Longevity science is constantly evolving, and a growing number of researchers have been exploring ways not only to increase lifespan, but to ensure that this time is lived with quality. Strategies involving diet, exercise, sleep, and stress management are proving to be as effective as, or more effective than, medications in addressing health problems related to aging.

Integrative Medicine is a model of medical care that combines conventional medicine with complementary, evidence-based practices, focusing on the patient as a whole: body, mind, and spirit. The goal is to treat not only the disease, but its deep-rooted causes, promoting lasting balance and well-being.

It uses therapies such as functional nutrition, herbal medicine, acupuncture, meditation, biohacking, personalized supplementation, mind-body therapies, and lifestyle adjustments, always grounded in scientific evidence and integrating the best of modern and traditional medicine. In addition, it prioritizes a more humanized physician-patient relationship, in which the patient plays an active role in the healing process.

Integrative medicine has its roots in the joining of ancient healing traditions, such as traditional Chinese medicine and Ayurveda, with the advances of Western medicine. In the 1970s and 1980s, it began gaining strength in the United States, driven by physicians who recognized the need for a broader approach to treating chronic diseases and improving patients' quality of life.

One important milestone was the creation of the Center for Integrative Medicine at the University of Arizona by Dr. Andrew Weil, author of 12 books, who helped consolidate this practice as a legitimate field within modern medicine. Now 83 years old, he teaches us that the happiness we all seek is within us, not outside us. Since then, various universities and healthcare centers around the world have adopted this approach, promoting more complete and effective treatments.

In Brazil, integrative medicine has been growing, especially after the inclusion of various integrative and complementary practices in the SUS, the Unified Health System, such as acupuncture, homeopathy, meditation, and herbal medicine. But it is we, the disruptive Brazilian doctors, who have been gaining more and more ground in the country every day. Tired of limited results, frustrated with the precarious healthcare system in one of the most corrupt countries in the world, Brazilian physicians today seek to promote integral health for their patients, providing measures for prevention, self-healing, and autonomy.

In the United States, integrative medicine is a well-established and growing field, adopted by hospitals, universities, and specialized clinics. Unlike the conventional approach focused solely on treating disease, Integrative Medicine in the United States emphasizes prevention, well-being, and personalized care, combining evidence-based medicine with complementary therapies. I cannot fail to mention The Institute for Functional Medicine, IFM, which offers programs and training for healthcare professionals.

The principles of integrative medicine include partnership between patient and physician in the healing process, the appropriate use of conventional and complementary methods, consideration of all the factors that influence health, well-being, and disease, the use of natural, effective, and less invasive therapeutic interventions, and the promotion of health and prevention of disease.

This approach seeks not only to treat symptoms, but also to address all the causes of a disease, taking into account biological, behavioral, psychosocial, and environmental influences in order to restore and maintain health over the long term.

The pursuit of longevity and full health, that is, when we are in balance with our physical, psychological, and spiritual conditions, has been a human goal for millennia. However, in recent decades, scientific discoveries and technological advances have opened the door to a new paradigm: biohacking. As I mentioned earlier, this revolutionary concept allows us, through personalized interventions, strategies, and technologies, to optimize our bodies and minds in order to achieve lasting well-being, greater vitality, and perhaps a longer, healthier life.

Throughout these pages, you will find accessible, evidence-based strategies to improve physical and mental performance, slow aging, and reach your body's maximum potential. Together, we will explore how small changes in lifestyle, combined with the power of scientific knowledge, can transform not only your health, but also your perception of aging, in other words, your healthspan.

Prepare yourself to challenge the limits of what you believe is possible for your body and mind. This is an invitation to take the reins of your health and optimize your path toward a longer, healthier, and fuller life.

This book sets out to be a practical guide for those who are ready to explore alternatives to the traditional model of health. I am both an advocate and a practitioner of the principles I will present throughout these chapters. This is not about abandoning conventional medicine, but about seeking an approach that places the patient at the center of their own health and well-being, giving them the tools to live healthier and longer lives..

CHAPTER 1

WHAT IS BIOHACKING?

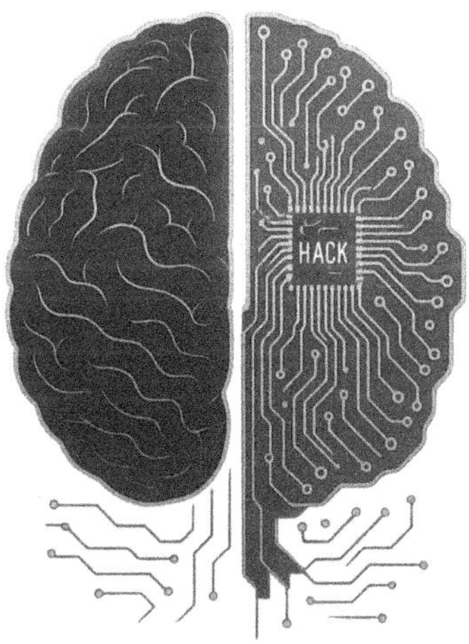

In the book's introduction, I spoke a little about biohacking, but we need to explore this term a bit further in order to understand what it encompasses and why it matters for our quality of life. So then, what is biohacking?

Biohacking is the practice of optimizing the functioning of the body and mind through lifestyle changes, nutrition, technologies, and even biological interventions. The goal is to improve health, longevity, and physical and mental performance in a strategic, science-based way.

There are different levels of biohacking, ranging from simple adjustments in diet and sleep to more advanced approaches, such as hormone therapies, personalized supplementation, controlled exposure to cold and heat, intermittent fasting, and even the use of technological devices for health monitoring, such as the Oura Ring, Whoop, and smartwatches. I will explore some of these approaches in the coming chapters.

Within integrative functional medicine, biohacking can be a great ally, because it focuses on personalizing treatment and seeking to optimize the body in a natural and preventive way.

The pursuit of optimized health and longevity is not limited to treating symptoms or following generic protocols. Instead, it requires a more personalized approach, one that considers the complexities and individual characteristics of each human being, and that is what I believe in. To achieve this level of precision, it is essential to integrate concepts from functional medicine, lifestyle medicine, and biohacking, three fields that, although distinct, converge toward a common goal: improving quality of life and extending health.

Functional Medicine:
Identifying and Treating the Underlying Causes

Functional medicine is an approach that seeks to understand the underlying causes of disease rather than simply treating symptoms. It examines the body as an integrated system, in which all organs and biological processes are interconnected. Through this lens, health problems are not viewed in isolation, but as manifestations of deeper imbalances within the body.

For example, a patient with digestive disorders, such as irritable bowel syndrome, may be facing imbalances in the gut microbiome, nutritional deficiencies, or even a chronic inflammatory response that can lead to depression. Instead of merely prescribing medication to relieve symptoms, or even to address the mood disorder, functional medicine seeks to identify what is causing these imbalances and to treat the patient holistically. This may involve dietary changes, the use of supplements, stress management, and often the use of advanced testing to measure biomarkers and understand the individual's health patterns.

Lifestyle Medicine:
The Power of Proven Changes

Lifestyle medicine, on the other hand, places great emphasis on prevention and on optimizing health through conscious daily choices. While conventional medicine often focuses on treatments for already established diseases, lifestyle medicine takes a proactive approach. It focuses on factors such as diet, physical activity, sleep, stress management, and social relationships, all recognized for their ability to deeply impact physical and mental health.

Studies have shown that simple lifestyle changes, such as adopting a nutrient-rich, balanced diet, exercising regularly, and improving sleep quality, can prevent and even reverse various chronic conditions, as demonstrated by the DiRECT study, published in The Lancet in 2016, which showed remission of type 2 diabetes, in addition to significantly reducing the incidence of hypertension and heart disease.

Instead of treating diseases after they manifest, lifestyle medicine seeks to keep the body in its ideal state of functioning, preventing imbalances from arising before they even appear.

Biohacking:

Personalizing and Optimizing Health Through Technology

While functional medicine and lifestyle medicine provide the foundation for optimizing health, biohacking introduces a new level of personalization. Biohacking, in its broadest sense, involves the use of technology and interventions to improve the body's biological, physical, and mental performance. The idea is to empower the individual to measure, understand, and adjust their own biology in order to achieve ideal health and well-being.

Personalization is the key here. With today's technologies, we can measure a wide range of biological data more precisely and accessibly than ever before. Tests such as DNA testing, gut microbiome analysis, and metabolomics, rings and wrist devices that assess body temperature, heart rate variability, and sleep, in addition to detailed bloodwork and continuous glucose or blood pressure monitoring, are just some of the tools being used to obtain a complete picture of the body. However, biohacking goes beyond simply collecting data. It focuses on using that information to optimize health in a way that is unique to each individual.

For example, instead of following general recommendations for "normal" cholesterol or glucose levels, a biohacker may seek to optimize these markers to ideal levels that support their specific health and longevity goals. This involves not only interpreting the data, but also implementing strategies such as intermittent fasting, personalized diets, or even the use of technologies such as brain stimulation to improve cognitive function. A recent example was a new study from the University of Surrey, published in PLOS Biology, showing exactly this. The study revealed that transcranial random noise stimulation, tRNS, when applied to the dorsolateral prefrontal cortex, dlPFC, can enhance mathematical learning in young adults with naturally weaker brain connectivity.

Biological Metrics and the New Health Paradigm

One of the main innovations these approaches have in common is the use of advanced biological metrics. Instead of relying on generic reference values, often derived from a sick or medicated population, functional medicine and biohacking seek to identify "optimal values" for the individual, values that indicate the body's ideal functioning. No more "normal" lab results in the first quartile, the metrics are different now.

When properly conducted, laboratory tests are not limited to comparing a patient's results with a population average, but should be used to identify patterns and discrepancies that may affect health over the long term. Functional medicine, for example, may measure hormone levels, such as cortisol or testosterone, more precisely, seeking not only to avoid disease, but to optimize hormonal function in order to ensure vibrant and lasting health. In biohacking, biomarkers of aging, such as telomerase or systemic inflammation levels, are analyzed to guide personalized interventions aimed at maximizing healthspan.

The integration of these technologies with lifestyle medicine practices creates a landscape in which the treatment and prevention of disease can be carried out in a far more precise, individualized, and proactive way. It is no longer about a one-size-fits-all standard, but about a health plan tailored to each individual's biological and metabolic needs.

The intersection of functional medicine, lifestyle medicine, and biohacking represents a more holistic and individualized model of care. By focusing on personalization and biological metrics, these approaches offer a more effective and sustainable path to health. With today's technologies, we can access deep data about our bodies, allowing a clearer understanding of our needs and the implementation of precise strategies to optimize our health and longevity.

I believe this is the future of medicine: a medicine that places the patient at the center of their own care, not merely as a recipient of generic treatments, but as an active agent in the pursuit of a longer, healthier, and fuller life.

As practical examples, I would like to share with you my morning ritual, a practice I have adopted and validated for some time:

1. Upon waking, I open the windows and get exposure to natural light;
2. I wash my mouth, brush my teeth, and scrape my tongue;
3. I drink 750 ml of water plus 2 grams of unrefined salt;

4. I do the Wim Hof breathing technique;
5. I take a cold shower;
6. I run according to a training plan or do strength training;
7. Post-workout infrared exposure, 15 minutes;
8. I take my morning shot;
9. I eat 5 pasture-raised eggs, boiled for 7 minutes in boiling water, and a cooked apple;
10. In the car, on the way to the office, I listen to worship music, declare, visualize, and pray;
11. I have my first tea of the day, usually matcha;
12. Smoothie with hydrolyzed protein plus personalized supplementation;
13. Lunch with family, non-negotiable;
14. In the afternoon, glasses that block blue light, caffeine prohibited;
15. At night, hot shower, socks, white noise;

Note:

1. I do not always do the breathing practice at home, sometimes I do it at the office. I can already hold an apnea for 2 minutes and 30 seconds.
2. While I am seated, I practice grounding in the office, where I use a grounding mat under the desk, which I bought on Amazon.

A powerful tool for recording and monitoring all the variables related to your health and performance, so as to optimize body and mind over time, is a biohacking journal, or even a simple checklist for beginners. It becomes a kind of data map, in which you collect information about your diet, exercise routine, sleep, biological metrics, use of technologies, and much more. The goal is to identify patterns, test new strategies, and continuously adjust your lifestyle, always with a focus on improving health and well-being.

Here is an example of how a biohacker's journal can be structured:

Biohacking Journal: How to Optimize the Body and Mind

Date: ____________

1. General State Upon Waking:

Energy:

1☐ 2☐ 3☐ 4☐ 5☐ 6☐ 7☐ 8☐ 9☐ 10☐

Mood:

1☐ 2☐ 3☐ 4☐ 5☐ 6☐ 7☐ 8☐ 9☐ 10☐

Sleep quality:

1☐ 2☐ 3☐ 4☐ 5☐ 6☐ 7☐ 8☐ 9☐ 10☐

Overall sense of well-being:

1☐ 2☐ 3☐ 4☐ 5☐ 6☐ 7☐ 8☐ 9☐ 10☐

Pain or discomfort: [Yes/No]

Yes☐ No☐

If so, what?

____

Notes: Any notable sensation upon waking

____

2. Morning Routine and Measurements

Hydration: Amount of water consumed

Sun exposure: Minutes spent in the sun

Exercise: Type and duration of exercise

Supplements taken: List of supplements and dosages

Intermittent fasting:

Yes ☐ No ☐

Fasting duration, if applicable

Technologies used: Use of devices such as glucose monitors, blue-light glasses, biofeedback devices, etc.

Health metrics: Monitoring of biological metrics, such as heart rate, heart rate variability, HRV, glucose, blood pressure, etc.

---

3. Nutrition

Meals:

Breakfast: What was consumed

Lunch: What was consumed

___

Dinner: What was consumed

___

Macros and micronutrients: Approximate amount of carbohydrates, proteins, fats, vitamins, and minerals

___

Relationship with food: How did you feel after the meals?

Satisfied ☐ Hungry ☐ Stable energy ☐

Notes: Did any specific food cause any notable effect?

___

4. Physical Activity

Type of exercise: Cardio, strength training, yoga, stretching, HIIT, etc.

___

Duration: Minutes

___

Intensity:

Low ☐ Medium ☐ High ☐

Post-exercise feeling: Tired, energized, sore muscles, etc.

___

Performance metrics: If applicable, such as weight lifted, distance covered, calories burned, etc.

___

Recovery: Rest time between sessions, recovery methods used, such as foam rolling, massage, sauna, ice immersion, etc.

___

5. Meditation and Mental Practices

Meditation: Time dedicated and type of meditation

___

Mindset and mental clarity: Sense of focus, anxiety, stress

___

Breathing exercises: Did you do breathing exercises?

Yes ☐ No ☐

Example: box breathing, diaphragmatic breathing

___

Neurofeedback or brain stimulation technologies: Use of devices such as Muse, Apollo, etc., feedback or changes noticed

___

Exposure to nature: Time outdoors and connection with the natural environment, grounding

___

6. Sleep Quality

Total sleep time: [Hours]

___

Sleep quality:

1☐ 2☐ 3☐ 4☐ 5☐ 6☐ 7☐ 8☐ 9☐ 10☐

Interruptions during sleep: [Number of times you woke up during the night]

1 ☐ 2 ☐ 3 ☐ 4 ☐ 5 ☐ 6 ☐ 7 ☐ 8 ☐ 9 ☐ 10 ☐ More ☐

Technologies used to monitor sleep: Devices such as Oura Ring, Fitbit, Garmin, etc.

___

Sleep ritual: Activities before sleeping, such as reading, relaxation, reduced blue light

___

7. Biological Measurements and Biohacking

Tests/Results: Results of recent tests such as bloodwork, hormones, gut microbiome analyses, etc.

___

Glucose: Average, spikes, or significant drops

___

HRV, Heart Rate Variability: Average, interpretation of the data

___

Blood pressure: Measurement and any noted changes

___

Other relevant parameters: Genetic tests, vitamin D levels, inflammation markers, etc.

___

Interventions made: Changes implemented to optimize results, such as dietary or supplementation adjustments

___

8. Feedback and Reflections

Perceived changes: New sensations or changes in health metrics

___

Biohacking goals: Progress in relation to established goals, such as improved cognitive performance, reduced body fat, increased energy

___

Lessons from the day: What worked well?

___

What can be improved? Any new strategy to be tested?

___

The biohacking journal is a dynamic tool that allows the biohacker to closely monitor their health and optimize their physical and mental condition. Each day brings an opportunity to adjust and test new strategies, based on real data and measurable results.

The goal is to transform the process of self-knowledge into a continuous system of improvement, in which the individual becomes the main person responsible for the pursuit of a healthier, longer life with greater performance.

This type of journal helps create a detailed view of how each aspect of the biohacker's life is affecting their body and mind. Over time, it becomes a valuable tool for identifying patterns, testing new strategies, and adjusting lifestyle more precisely.

Task:

- Create a biohacking journal, according to the example mentioned, so that you can track your progress and have an overall view of your health.

- Define and write down three areas of your health that you want to improve over the next 30 days:

____

____

____

____

"Biohacking is the process of self-discovery and optimization of the human body using science, technology, and practical experimentation to achieve maximum physical, mental, and emotional performance." Ben Greenfield, Boundless: Upgrade Your Brain, Optimize Your Body & Defy Aging, 2020.

CHAPTER 2

ICE IMMERSION, THE POWER OF CRYOTHERAPY

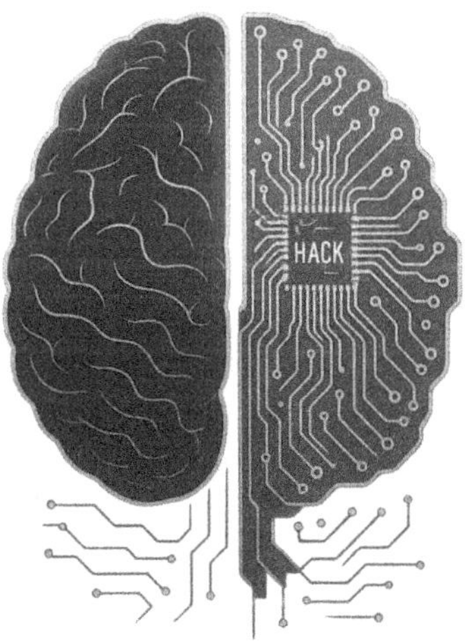

Have you ever heard about the incredible benefits of ice baths or cryotherapy? If you are still not convinced about stepping into a freezing tub, perhaps this chapter and my experience will change your mind. Science has shown that cold is not just uncomfortable, it is powerful. It can improve your mood, speed up your metabolism, strengthen your mind, and even help prevent degenerative diseases such as Alzheimer's.

In recent years, ice immersion has become increasingly popular as a therapeutic practice, especially in the world of sports and wellness. Elite athletes, people engaged in intense physical activity, and even those seeking an overall boost in health have been turning to this technique, which involves submerging the body in cold water, usually between 0 and 10°C, for controlled periods.

The idea of using cold as a form of treatment is not new. Throughout history, various cultures have used ice and cold water as ways to relieve pain and injuries. In Ancient Greece, for example, the physician Hippocrates already advocated the use of ice to heal wounds and inflammation. However, it was only in recent decades that ice immersion became established as a scientifically proven technique for accelerating muscle recovery, reducing inflammation, and even improving psychological well-being.

Exposure to cold, especially through ice baths or cryotherapy, has received growing attention because of its significant effects on the human body. Far from being merely a physical challenge, intentional contact with cold triggers a series of highly beneficial hormonal, neurological, and metabolic responses, with applications ranging from improved physical performance to the prevention of neurodegenerative diseases. This type of stimulus, although uncomfortable at first, represents a powerful inducer of adaptations that strengthen both body and mind.

One of the most notable effects of exposure to ice is the marked increase in neurotransmitters such as dopamine and norepinephrine. Norepinephrine, released in large amounts during extreme cold, is directly related to heightened alertness, increased focus, and reduced inflammation. Dopamine, known as the neurotransmitter of motivation and pleasure, can have its levels increased by as much as 250% after just 20 seconds in 4°C water, an effect comparable to that of psychoactive substances, yet achieved naturally. This neurochemical response not only improves mood and energy, but also contributes to long-term mental well-being.

In addition to its neurochemical effects, exposure to cold strongly stimulates mitochondrial activity, especially through the activation of brown fat. Unlike white fat, which is responsible only for energy storage, brown fat has a high density of mitochondria, the body's power plants. Cells with high energy demand can contain up to 10,000 mitochondria. Mitochondria account for about 5% of body weight, and increasing their number, size, and activity is crucial for optimized health. Ice exposure contributes to this by indirectly stimulating mitochondrial biogenesis through powerful adaptive mechanisms. Their primary function is energy production, ATP, and secondarily heat production. This process, called thermogenesis, not only increases energy expenditure at rest, but also enhances fat burning and improves insulin sensitivity. Thus, ice immersion becomes a powerful ally in fighting obesity and metabolic diseases, activating the browning process through the expression of UCP1, a phenomenon in which white adipose tissue, WAT, acquires characteristics of brown adipose tissue, BAT, which is extremely rich in mitochondria.

Interestingly, populations traditionally exposed to cold environments, such as Eskimos, or Inuit, provide empirical evidence of these benefits. These peoples have a greater proportion of brown fat and specific metabolic adaptations that allow them to withstand intense cold without harm to their health. Even with highly caloric, high-fat diets, they maintain low rates of cardiovascular and metabolic diseases, probably thanks to the constant thermoregulation required by their environment.

Another essential element in this process is irisin, a hormone released by the muscles both during physical exercise and during exposure to cold. Irisin plays a fundamental role in converting white fat into brown fat and is associated with improved metabolic function, increased insulin sensitivity, and neuroprotection. Recent studies have highlighted the importance of this hormone, including a 2021 study by Robert Sallis and colleagues in the British Journal of Sports Medicine, which used data from the Kaiser Permanente Southern California health system. Low levels of irisin were associated with up to a 2.5-fold increase in the risk of death from the disease when active individuals were compared with sedentary ones, possibly due to the anti-inflammatory role of this substance, helping control the inflammatory cytokine storm in COVID-19 and regulating the immune system.

The effects of exposure to cold are not limited to the body. In the brain, the combination of stimuli such as increased norepinephrine and irisin contributes to the release of Brain-Derived Neurotrophic Factor, BDNF, a protein essential for neurogenesis, that is, the formation of new neurons. BDNF is directly linked to improved memory, learning, and brain plasticity, and is considered a protective factor against diseases such as Alzheimer's and Parkinson's. By stimulating its production, the regular practice of cryotherapy also emerges as an ally in preserving cognitive health and preventing dementia.

Therefore, cold, far from being merely a discomfort to be avoided, can be understood as a natural resource of high therapeutic value. Its effects are broad and demonstrably effective, from metabolic activation to hormonal modulation, from strengthening the immune system to neuronal regeneration. Just as Eskimos adapted to the frozen environment as a means of survival, today we can use this natural stressor intentionally and in a controlled way to achieve higher levels of health, performance, and resilience.

But how exactly does ice immersion work? When the body is exposed to intense cold, it initiates a series of physiological reactions designed to minimize the damage caused by thermal stress. Heat shock proteins, HSPs, are activated, helping repair damaged cells and reduce inflammation. Ice immersion also improves blood circulation, increasing the supply of oxygen and nutrients to muscles and tissues, which favors faster recovery.

My journey with ice began as part of my preparation to take part in a half marathon, after having faced nine injuries and several treatments, including the use of morphine, PRP injections, laser, and ozone therapy, the most important being a near rupture of my Achilles tendon. Since then, the results obtained through this practice have been impressive and transformative, both physically and mentally.

Personally, I adopt this technique as part of my preparation routine for immersions in ice tubs, which has contributed significantly to my performance in physical activities. The process begins with the Wim Hof breathing practice, which I do in three apnea rounds: 30 seconds in the first, 1 minute in the second, and 1 minute and 30 seconds in the third. This sequence promotes alkalinization of blood pH and intense oxygenation of tissues and organs, which prepares the body effectively for the thermal stress that will follow.

If you have never heard of the Wim Hof breathing technique, it is worth learning a little about it. It was developed by the Dutch athlete of the same name, also known as "The Iceman," and has gained recognition for its effectiveness in improving physical and mental health through a combination of conscious breathing, cold exposure, and mind control. The technique is based on cryotherapy, which means remaining in an extremely cold environment for a set period of time. According to Wim, the method is the union of cold, breathing, and meditation. The main benefits of this practice include increased energy, reduced stress, strengthening of the immune system, and the development of physical and mental endurance. I recommend watching episode two of the series The Goop Lab with Gwyneth Paltrow, in which Wim Hof appears.

After the breathing rounds mentioned above, I enter the ice tub and remain there for 2 to 7 minutes, depending on my condition that day. During immersion, I continue with a specific breathing pattern: I inhale deeply, hold the air for a few seconds, and exhale slowly as if I were blowing through a straw. This technique helps not only maintain emotional control, but also preserve body heat, slowing the loss of internal temperature and bringing a sense that time passes more quickly. After all, a long inhale, a pause, and a slow exhale make two minutes feel like 30 seconds. One of the signs I use to determine the right time to get out of the tub is when my jaw begins to shake. For me, this is a clear sign that I have reached my limit and that insisting beyond that point would no longer be beneficial; believe me, it is real.

The initial sensation when entering the tub is usually one of desperation. It is precisely at that moment that breathing and self-control become essential. Learning to deal with this sensation develops what I call "mental callusing," expanding physical and emotional endurance, increasing resilience, and reducing procrastination. Just as callused hands become stronger through manual labor, the mind becomes more resilient when voluntarily exposed to controlled stress, allowing a person to go through real stress with greater wisdom and lightness. A person who submits to ice immersion begins to respond better in situations of pressure and rapid decision-making, both at work and in personal life. This type of physiological stress is known as hormesis, the body's positive adaptation to adverse stimuli. This metabolic activation has been directly reflected in improvements in my health and energy.

Contrast therapy is also part of my routine: I like to alternate between a dry sauna and an ice tub. I usually stay in the dry sauna for about 15 minutes, which I prefer because it does not release steam with possible contaminants such as chlorine, trihalomethanes , or THMs, which are formed when chlorine added to water reacts with decomposing organic matter, and which may be carcinogenic and hepatotoxic, as well as fluoride and medication residues, and then I do the ice immersion, for times ranging between 2 and 10 minutes according to my tolerance on that day. The combination of hyperthermia, increased body temperature in the sauna, and hypothermia, cooling in the ice, generates extremely beneficial effects for the body, promoting greater muscle recovery, improved circulation, and balance of the autonomic nervous system.

It is important to remember that each individual perceives cold differently. Some people may need gloves or thermal rubber socks to protect more sensitive extremities. Adaptation should be done progressively and consciously, respecting the limits of one's own body.

I like to say that challenges break us out of inertia, lead us into a virtuous cycle, help us grow and develop, and awaken our personal power. Whenever I challenge myself, I not only leave my comfort zone, but also prove to myself that the greater the strength of my mindset, the smaller the power of the people and situations that try to bring me down.

As I mentioned earlier, during ice immersion our bodies produce 540% more norepinephrine and 300% more dopamine.

Studies show that this is excellent for fighting depression and anxiety. In addition, the liver releases cold shock proteins that help reduce oxidative stress caused by free radicals in the blood and quadruple the rate of protein synthesis that favors muscle repair.

After my first 21-kilometer run, I immersed myself in ice for 5 minutes at a temperature of zero degrees. This helped reduce the inflammation generated by acute physical stress and contributed to the reprogramming of my mind and the detoxification of my body.

Studies show that ice immersion also increases male fertility, because there is cooling and a low temperature in the testicles, stimulating sperm production.

Historically, cryotherapy goes back centuries. However, its therapeutic use became more prevalent in the late twentieth century, especially in the context of muscle recovery and sports injuries. Today, it is widely applied for reducing inflammation, relieving muscle pain, recovering from injuries, and even for aesthetic purposes, such as skin rejuvenation.

As we already know, the use of cold for therapeutic treatments goes back to Ancient Greece, with Hippocrates mentioning the use of ice to relieve inflammation and wounds. However, the modern form of cryotherapy, especially immersion in cold water, gained popularity among professional athletes in the 1970s, with a significant increase in its use after the development of cryotherapy chambers in the 1980s.

During immersion, the body goes through a series of physiological responses. The first is vasoconstriction, in other words, the narrowing of blood vessels, which reduces blood flow to the muscles and other parts of the body. This helps reduce inflammation and pain. After immersion, when the body returns to normal temperature, vasodilation occurs, which increases blood flow and promotes recovery and tissue repair.

At first, people generally experience a sensation of thermal shock, followed by a feeling of numbness and progressive pain relief. In the beginning, the skin becomes very cold, and discomfort may occur due to the impact of the cold. However, after a few minutes, the body adapts to the temperature and sensations of pain begin to diminish. When immersion ends, the muscles may feel more relaxed, and there is a feeling of renewal and well-being.

There are demonstrably many benefits of cryotherapy and ice immersion for the body, and I have experienced this myself. I will list some of them below:

1. Increased dopamine;
2. Release of norepinephrine and adrenaline;
3. Anti-inflammatory effect;
4. Optimizes sleep;
5. Favors thermogenesis and tissue browning;
6. Increased irisin;
7. Improves cardiovascular health;
8. Improves muscle recovery;
9. Resilience to stress;
10. Enhancement of the immune system;
11. Increased metabolism;
12. Improves adaptation to abrupt temperature changes.

This practice has also become widespread among elite athletes, such as soccer players, runners, and fighters, who frequently use cryotherapy as part of their recovery routine. Cold therapy not only accelerates recovery after intense training and competition, but also helps reduce the possibility of future injuries, making it an essential tool for athletes seeking to maintain high performance.

Several studies have demonstrated the effectiveness of cryotherapy in muscle recovery and pain reduction. Research shows that ice immersion can significantly decrease markers of inflammation, such as cytokines, cytokines are proteins or glycoproteins that act as cellular messengers, helping control the body's immune response, in addition to promoting faster muscle regeneration. However, the scientific community still debates the best protocol to optimize the benefits, including the duration and frequency of immersion.

Although cryotherapy is generally safe for most people, there are some contraindications. People with cardiovascular disease, severe hypertension, or circulatory problems such as Raynaud's syndrome should avoid ice immersion. People with skin diseases or cold allergies may have adverse reactions to the treatment.

If poorly applied, cryotherapy can cause harm. Prolonged exposure to cold can result in hypothermia, bradycardia, frostbite, and nerve damage. For this reason, it is essential to follow safety protocols supervised by qualified professionals to avoid these risks.

Although it is best known for its benefits to athletes, cryotherapy can also be advantageous for people seeking to improve their general well-being. Ice immersion can be an effective way to combat daily stress, improve sleep quality, and even promote skin health due to increased circulation and reduced inflammation.

The future of cryotherapy looks promising, with technological innovations ranging from temperature-controlled cryotherapy chambers to portable devices that offer targeted cold treatments. These new approaches may make cryotherapy more accessible and effective, allowing more people to benefit from its effects.

Cryotherapy, especially ice immersion, offers a series of powerful benefits for body and mind, as we have seen. By promoting muscle recovery, reducing inflammation, and improving mental well-being, it establishes itself as an effective therapy for a wide range of people, from elite athletes to those seeking to improve their quality of life. However, like any treatment, it is important to practice it responsibly, respecting professional guidance and the body's individual needs.

Stimulating the Expression of Heat Shock Proteins, HSPs:

What Are Heat Shock Proteins, HSPs?

Heat shock proteins, HSPs, are a group of proteins produced by cells in response to physical stress, such as exposure to extreme temperatures, heat or cold, radiation, toxins, or inflammation. They play a crucial role in protecting cells, helping repair damaged proteins and preventing cellular collapse.

These proteins help maintain cellular homeostasis and ensure the integrity of cells under adverse conditions. In response to thermal stresses, such as exposure to cold, the body increases the production of HSPs to protect its cells and promote repair processes.

The best-known HSPs include HSP70, which is one of the most studied because of its role in several biological functions, including cellular recovery, reduction of oxidative damage, and strengthening of the immune system.

How Does Cryotherapy Stimulate HSP Expression?

Cryotherapy, especially ice immersion, can be an effective way to stimulate the expression of heat shock proteins. When the body is exposed to intense cold, it enters a state of controlled stress, which activates the production of HSPs. This occurs because cells perceive the thermal stress and initiate a protective process to prevent damage. Repeated exposure to cold can increase the body's ability to express HSPs more efficiently and in greater quantity, helping improve the cells' resistance to stress.

Studies have shown that exposure to cold can induce the production of HSPs, promoting improved cellular repair and muscle recovery after injuries or intense exertion. This increase in HSPs has been linked to increased cellular longevity, strengthening of the immune system, and prevention of neurodegenerative diseases.

If you have not yet tried it and would like to incorporate cold showers, cryotherapy chambers, and gradual exposure to cold into your routine, I am going to give you a few tips:

Ice tubs, my favorite method: immersion in cold water is one of the most accessible ways to activate HSPs.. To incorporate this into your routine, you can follow these tips:

- Ideal temperature: the water temperature should be between 0°C and 15°C to be effective in activating HSPs. Respect safety and individual progression.
- Duration: start with 1 to 3 minutes and gradually increase as your body becomes accustomed to the cold. The goal is to activate thermal stress without causing harm.
- Frequency: for maximum benefits, it is recommended to do immersion 2 to 3 times per week. It may be especially interesting to do this after intense training, when the body needs muscle recovery.
- Precautions: begin with short exposure and avoid prolonged immersion. If you feel you are becoming too uncomfortable, it is important to get out of the water immediately.

Cryo Chambers: cryotherapy chambers offer a controlled extreme-cold experience and are a more effective way to induce HSP production. These chambers reach much lower temperatures, from -100°C to -150°C, and provide cold exposure for a short period, usually between 2 and 3 minutes. The use of these chambers has several benefits:

- Access to lower temperatures: this can induce a more intense thermal response, stimulating greater HSP production.
- Rapid benefits: because of the intensity of the cold, cryotherapy offers a more immediate impact on the body, accelerating recovery and the production of heat shock proteins.
- Muscle recovery: high-level athletes and people seeking to improve their physical performance use these chambers to reduce muscle recovery time, in addition to benefiting the immune system and metabolism.

Gradual Exposure to Cold: gradual exposure to cold is an effective way to accustom the body to thermal stress, promoting benefits without causing major discomfort or risks. Some ways to do this include:

- Progressive cold showers: start with warm water and gradually lower the temperature during the shower, ending the last 30 seconds with cold water. This can preferably be done every day or every other day.
- Exposure to cold throughout the day: you can incorporate small doses of cold, such as walking outdoors in lower temperatures, wearing lighter clothes in cold environments, or practicing controlled breathing in cold settings, such as the Wim Hof technique.

Studies suggest that stimulating heat shock proteins can have beneficial effects on cellular longevity and on preventing age-related diseases. HSPs help to:

Reduce cellular damage and oxidative stress, factors associated with premature aging and the development of chronic diseases such as Alzheimer's and Parkinson's.

Increase resistance to stress: HSP production can also help the body better resist environmental stress, promoting healthy aging.

Promote cellular repair: by improving the body's ability to repair damaged cells, cryotherapy can help maintain health over the long term.

Incorporating cryotherapy and exposure to cold into the daily routine can be an excellent way to stress the body positively, activating the production of heat shock proteins, HSPs, and providing significant benefits for muscle recovery, athletic performance, and cellular longevity.

Whether through cold showers, ice tubs, cryo chambers, or gradual exposure, the advantages of cold for the body are numerous, and the science behind these practices is increasingly recognized. However, like any practice, it is important to begin gradually and always with proper guidance, ensuring safety and the effectiveness of long-term benefits.

Putting It Into Practice:

Try a 30-second cold shower and gradually increase it to 2 minutes over time.

Notice how you feel before, during, and after the shower.

CHAPTER 3

PRACTICAL GUIDE TO SUPPLEMENTATION AND BENEFITS

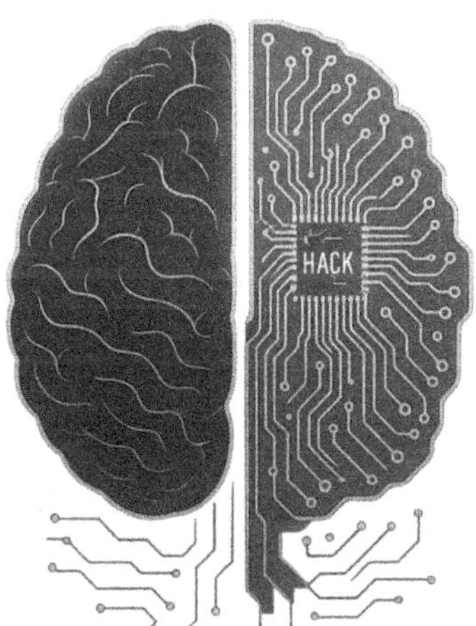

Nowadays, the pursuit of a healthy life and improved physical and mental performance is at the center of attention for many people. Among the various tools that help achieve these goals, dietary supplementation has become an increasingly popular resource, and today we find everything, both high quality and poor-quality supplements: some that work, some that make no difference, some with artificial coloring, some with clean labels, some expensive, and some cheap. With our hectic lives, in which we opt for fast food, with soil too poor in nutrients to transfer them to food and meet all the body's nutritional needs. Especially when we are seeking results that are simple, fast, and effective, whether in training, recovery, or daily life, supplementation becomes necessary.

Although dietary supplements do not replace a balanced diet, they are a powerful complement for correcting nutritional deficiencies, enhancing results, and even improving overall health. From proteins that help with muscle recovery to vitamins and minerals that keep the body functioning optimally, supplementation has been an important ally for those seeking to improve performance, increase energy, or achieve long-term goals.

This chapter will be a practical guide to supplementation, detailing the types of supplements, how to choose the one most appropriate for your specific needs, and the benefits each one can provide. The key to using supplementation effectively lies in understanding how it can be integrated intelligently into your routine, making the most of its properties without risking excess or improper use.

"Vitamin supplementation has been widely used to correct nutritional deficiencies, improve health outcomes, and optimize physiological functions, especially in individuals with specific health needs or restrictive diets." (Souza & Silva, 2018)

We live in an age in which an abundance of food does not guarantee health. The table is full, but the plate is poor. Modern eating is often monotonous, ultra-processed, and lacking in essential nutrients. This is made worse by nutrient-depleted soils, excessive use of pesticides, and a routine that makes adequate sun exposure difficult. Supplementing, therefore, is not a luxury. It is a strategy. But it must be done intelligently, respecting bio-individuality and the synergy among nutrients.

Brazilian and American soils, for example, show different fertility patterns. In Brazil, excess aluminum and natural acidity demand constant correction. In the United States, despite mechanization and large-scale fertilization, studies show a decline in the nutritional content of food since the 1950s.

In addition, pesticide use affects the soil microbiota and, consequently, the nutritional quality of food. A plant that does not find minerals in the soil cannot transfer them to the food. And the human being who consumes that deficient food becomes ill.

The choice of supplements we should take depends on several factors, such as diet, personal goals, lifestyle, and the body's individual needs. However, some supplements are widely recommended because of their well-documented functions and proven health benefits, especially when there are nutritional deficiencies or specific goals to be achieved.

But not every supplement is safe. Many capsules are formulated with artificial colorings, titanium dioxide, aluminum hydroxide, preservatives, and even nanoparticles. These additives may be toxic and cause more harm than benefit in the long run.

We know today that toxic metals and artificial colorings are co-responsible for countless conditions such as autism, cancer, and ADHD, so I would not recommend spending a lifetime taking capsules with these chemical products.

That is why the source laboratory matters. Inform yourself, check purity tests, stability, quality certifications, traceability, and whether there are bioavailability tests, as required by law in Brazil. Your doctor may also indicate laboratories he or she trusts.

In the biochemistry of the human body, nothing acts in isolation. Nutrients do not work alone, they connect, collaborate, compete, or even cancel one another out. It is important to understand these interactions in order to build a supplementation strategy that is truly effective and safe. Many times, the expected effects of a supplement do not appear not because the nutrient failed, but because a cofactor is absent or because it is competing with another mineral. Let me explain a little better.

The World Health Organization, WHO, warns of a problem that is increasingly common on a global scale: chronic vitamin and mineral deficiency, even in populations that consume excess calories. In clinical practice, doctors like me, who order broader testing, often find obese patients who are undernourished at the micronutrient level. This phenomenon is known as "hidden hunger," a type of malnutrition that, although it does not necessarily appear as extreme thinness, compromises health at deep levels. It is common to see people who are overweight or obese presenting severe nutritional deficiencies. They are overfed in caloric terms, but undernourished in terms of essential micronutrients.

In this context, supplementation can be a valuable tool, but it must be carried out with caution and intelligence. In functional nutrition, the principle that prevails is that less is more. Indiscriminate supplementation, without individualized assessment, can generate important metabolic imbalances, especially because many minerals compete with one another in absorption and use by the body. For example, excess zinc can reduce copper absorption, and high doses of iron can interfere with magnesium assimilation.

Understanding the physiological mechanisms behind supplementation is essential. Enough with compounded formulas or products with dozens of compounds in one capsule. These are the kinds of prescriptions and over-the counter supplements that generate simplistic comments on the subject. You have probably heard that taking supplements is just making expensive urine, perhaps because some supplements that exceed therapeutic limits have made your urine fluorescent, as though you were taking kryptonite. Nutrient replacement must be strategic, based on clinical signs, laboratory tests, and knowledge about micronutrient interactions. Supplementing with purpose, not because of trends or generalizations, is the safest and most effective path to promoting health, performance, and longevity.

A classic example of this synergy is vitamin D, known for its fundamental role in calcium regulation. However, for vitamin D to be activated and fully perform its function, it depends on the presence of magnesium and retinol. Without magnesium and sufficient vitamin A, the body cannot absorb and convert vitamin D into its active form, calcitriol, impairing not only calcium absorption but also immune and hormonal processes.

Another crucial nutrient in this picture is vitamin K2, often neglected. It acts like a kind of calcium GPS, directing calcium to the bones and teeth, where it is needed, and preventing its deposition in soft tissues such as arteries and kidneys. The absence of K2, especially in people who supplement large amounts of vitamin D and calcium, may increase the risk of atherosclerosis and unwanted calcifications. In addition, vitamin K2 MK7 stabilizes atherosclerotic plaque, preventing its development.

The relationship between zinc and copper also deserves attention. These two minerals directly compete for intestinal absorption, and isolated zinc supplementation over long periods may lead to copper deficiency, which can cause anemia, lowered immunity, and even neurological changes. For this reason, in many cases, it is recommended to respect the proportion between them or alternate supplementation, always based on test results. For every 10 mg of zinc there should be 1 mg of copper. The proportion is important so that there is homeostasis between zinc and copper, and it is important to take them away from iron and calcium, since they compete for absorption.

Another important point is the competition between iron and calcium. Both use the same absorption channels in the intestine, and when they are consumed together, especially in large amounts, one can inhibit the absorption of the other. For that reason, the ideal is to consume iron and calcium supplements at different times of day. I would recommend zinc and copper at breakfast, iron with vitamin C at lunch, and calcium at night, but personalized medical assessment is what will guide the best approach.

It is also worth highlighting the synergistic action between iron and vitamin C. Vitamin C increases the bioavailability of non-heme iron, found in plant sources, helping prevent and treat deficiency states, especially in pregnant women and vegetarians. Just one source of vitamin C, such as acerola, orange, or lemon, can significantly improve the absorption of iron present in a meal.

All these examples show that supplementation should not be done blindly, with an isolated approach or based on internet trends. It is necessary to understand the biochemical context, the antagonisms, the synergies, and the safe doses. The human body is an interdependent network of systems, and each nutrient needs the other for the machinery of health to function perfectly. Therefore, it is essential that you talk with your trusted physician. Do not supplement on your own because you run a great risk of doing it in a way that prevents you from properly benefiting from the supplements you use.

Although supplementation can be a powerful ally for health, not every supplement is harmless. When it is done indiscriminately, without individual assessment and without considering genetic variants or specific contexts, it can do more harm than good.

A classic and concerning example is synthetic folic acid, widely used in supplements for pregnant women. Although folic acid is fundamental for fetal neural tube formation and the prevention of congenital malformations, not everyone is able to metabolize this synthetic form efficiently. It is estimated that up to 40 to 60% of the population has some degree of polymorphism in the MTHFR gene, methylenetetrahydrofolate reductase, which is responsible for converting folic acid into its active form, methylfolate. Since my wife and I now know our genetic parameters, we already supplement with methylfolate, L-5-MTHF, in ourselves and our children.

In people with this polymorphism, synthetic folic acid can accumulate in the body, leading to liver overload and even neurotoxic effects. Instead of protection, the supplement may increase the risk of neurological dysfunctions, behavioral changes, and, according to some emerging studies, a potential association with autism spectrum disorders in the children of pregnant women who used excessive amounts of synthetic folic acid.

This reality requires a change of paradigm. It is not enough to prescribe folic acid because that is how it has always been done. It is necessary to look at the individual, investigate possible genetic variants, and, when necessary, choose bioactive forms such as methylfolate, L-5-MTHF, which already comes ready for use by the body.

And folic acid is only one of many examples. Iron supplements, for example, can cause constipation, oxidative stress, and even imbalances in the intestinal microbiota when used in excess or without real need. Common multivitamins, often filled with artificial colors, preservatives, titanium dioxide, aluminum, magnesium stearate, and nanoparticles, may compromise intestinal function and overload the liver and kidneys over time.

It is known that many products on the market do not undergo bioavailability testing, meaning the body cannot even absorb what is being ingested. A person thinks they are taking care of themselves, when in fact they are merely accumulating inactive or toxic compounds.

That is why supplementing correctly is an art that requires science, personalization, and responsibility. It is not enough to choose what is fashionable or what the neighbor is taking. It is necessary to understand the chemical forms of nutrients, the right time to use them, the interactions with other nutrients, and, above all, what is truly lacking in the body.

One of the biggest mistakes in supplementation is treating the human body as a standardized and static system. In reality, we are dynamic organisms, influenced by genetic, environmental, emotional, and dietary factors. For that reason, individualized assessment is the first step in any effective supplementation plan. Blood and saliva laboratory tests, combined with the patient's clinical history and lifestyle, help map deficiencies, excesses, and specific needs. What works for one person may not work for another, and what is good today may not be necessary tomorrow.

It is essential to respect the body's natural rhythm. Many substances, especially antioxidants such as curcumin, quercetin, and propolis, exert beneficial effects when used strategically, but they can become pro-oxidants if used excessively or continuously. The ideal is to adopt a rotating and cyclical supplementation scheme, for example, using one antioxidant for three months, taking a break, and starting another, always observing the body's response and reevaluating as needed. In my clinical practice, I use patented formulas such as Cureit, curcumin, GlucoVantage, berberine, and Resvitec, resveratrol, which are highly bioavailable, stable, and safe and, at the appropriate dose, protect the body against hepato-metabolic overload and keep internal antioxidant systems in balance during a cyclical regimen.

Another frequently ignored aspect is the way nutrients are absorbed. Fat-soluble vitamins, A, D, E, and K, need fat to be properly absorbed in the intestine. Supplementing them without ingesting a healthy source of fat, such as olive oil, egg yolks, or coconut oil, may compromise their effectiveness. On the other hand, water-soluble vitamins, such as vitamin C and the B complex, dissolve in water and the excess is eliminated in the urine. That gave rise to the famous idea that supplementing is just making expensive urine. Although there is truth in that statement, it should not be used as an argument to dismiss supplementation. Waste occurs when people supplement without criteria, without adequate dosage, and without real need, as stated earlier.

Therefore, supplementing intelligently is much more than taking capsules daily. It is observing, understanding, adjusting, and respecting the body's natural processes. It is giving the body what it needs, at the right time and in the right form. And above all, it is remembering that health is balance, not excess.

Studies show that nutritional deficiency compromises vaccine response. A 1980 study already pointed to the relationship between malnutrition and the absence of antibodies. Many elderly people vaccinated against COVID-19 did not develop an effective response because of deficiencies in selenium, vitamin E, B-complex vitamins, and zinc.

Without nutritional substrate, there is no immune system that can function properly.

Another point worth discussing is fertility. We are living in an age in which human fertility is declining. Couples are facing more and more difficulty conceiving, and when they do succeed, many babies come into the world already exposed to a nutritionally impoverished environment. We are facing a generation of infertility, and the environmental and nutritional context plays a central role in this scenario. Integrative practices, and especially precision nutrition, can make the dream of becoming a mother a reality. At the Melo Institute of Integrative Medicine, we have achieved major results in preconception programs. Our genius babies, as I nickname them, continue to arrive, healthy, and into homes of couples who were already exhausted by injections, IVF treatments, and frustrated attempts.

Soils are increasingly poor, the use of pesticides and fertilizers affects the microbiota and the nutritional density of foods, and the modern diet, based on ultra-processed products, is poor in vitamins, minerals, and antioxidants. This compromises not only fertility, but also intrauterine health, which is the foundation of the baby's future health. According to a comparative study published in 2004 in the Journal of the American College of Nutrition, which analyzed 43 cultivars of vegetables and fruits in the United States between 1950 and 1999, the authors found significant declines in protein content, minus 6%, calcium, minus 16%, iron, minus 15%, riboflavin, B2, minus 38%, and ascorbic acid, minus 20%.

During pregnancy, the demand for nutrients increases significantly, and one aspect rarely discussed is that placentas of boys and girls behave differently.

These differences involve everything from glucose metabolism to gene expression and hormonal response.

Research shows that pregnancies with boys are associated with a higher risk of gestational diabetes, possibly because of the influence of placental lactogenic hormones, which alter maternal insulin sensitivity.

In light of this, an important reflection arises: should mothers of boys have specific nutritional strategies and supplementation, adjusted to the metabolic profile of the male placenta, to better prevent the risk of gestational diabetes? This is where intelligent supplementation becomes a form of biological shielding, not only to protect the mother, but to ensure that the baby receives everything needed to develop with physical and neurological health.

Nutrients such as iron, zinc, iodine, choline, vitamin D, B12, DHA fatty acid, and methylfolate are absolutely essential in this process. Deficiency in any one of them can impair brain formation, increase the risk of premature birth, preeclampsia, and even neurodevelopmental disorders such as autism. It is known that the market now offers various types of encapsulated supplement formulas for support from preconception through the postpartum period.

Studies already show a concerning correlation: pregnant women with iron deficiency in the first trimester have a greater risk of having children with autism spectrum disorder, ASD. Methylfolate deficiency, as mentioned earlier, also enters this picture, further worsening the risks in pregnant women with mutations in the MTHFR gene. It is very important not to confuse folic acid with methylfolate. Failure to distinguish between them may put the embryonic process and fetal development at risk in cases of incorrect supplementation.

Today, 1 in every 40 live births is diagnosed with ASD, autism spectrum disorder, a number that continues to grow. This is not explained solely by better diagnosis, but by a sum of environmental, dietary, genetic, and epigenetic factors, all directly linked to the mother's nutrition before and during pregnancy, in addition to the obvious, indiscriminate vaccination. In 1984, the year I was born, the prevalence of children diagnosed with autism spectrum disorder, ASD, was estimated at 1 in every 2,000 live births.

For that reason, it is fundamental to expose this pain and open a dialogue with women who are planning to become pregnant or are already pregnant. Supplementing correctly, with professional guidance, with active vitamin forms, with prior testing and laboratory follow-up, can be a turning point.

Supplementing is not a luxury, it is an investment in the health of the next generation. And perinatal nutrition is one of the most important pillars for breaking cycles of disease and cognitive, immune, and metabolic dysfunction in the coming decades.

Supplementation, when carried out in a guided and evidence-based way, can be a powerful tool for filling nutritional gaps, optimizing metabolic functions, and preventing disease. Next, I want to talk about the most recommended supplements, according to the scientific literature and clinical practice, with their main benefits and points of attention.

Magnesium is the mineral of metabolic vitality because it is involved in more than 600 enzymatic reactions in the body, yet 75% of people do not consume enough of it. Without it, critical biochemical processes are turned off. The benefits of magnesium are endless. It acts in energy production, ATP, glucose regulation, muscle function, cardiovascular health, the nervous system, and sleep quality. It is indicated for stress control, cramps, insomnia, constipation, premenstrual syndrome, and insulin resistance. There are several forms of magnesium, glycinate and threonate are good for the brain, citrate for the intestines, malate for energy.

What is fascinating about magnesium is that it follows a daily rhythm in your body. It is lower in the morning and higher at night. That is why supplementing at night works better, because it supports your natural cycle.

Vitamin D3 plus K2 form an inseparable duo for bones, immunity, and longevity. Vitamin D, through the VDR receptor, has a broad transcriptional epigenetic impact, regulating hundreds to thousands of genes related to the immune system and inflammation, the cell cycle and apoptosis, and energy metabolism. In addition, it extraordinarily helps with calcium absorption, which will act in synergy with vitamin K2.

Vitamin K2, in turn, directs that calcium to the bones, preventing its deposition in the arteries, preventing calcification, helping mental health, increasing metabolism, improving intestinal health, and even increasing testosterone. It is fundamental for immunity, strong bones, and cardiovascular prevention. It should be associated with magnesium and healthy fats for better absorption. Supplementing D3 without K2 may increase the risk of atherosclerosis. Unlike most doctors and commercial brands that generally associate vitamin K2 MK7 with vitamin D, in my clinical practice I suggest that, when possible, we use vitamin K2 MK4 as the best option after individualizing the clinical case.

Vitamin K2 MK4 is superior in clinical contexts such as advanced osteoporosis, cancer, male infertility, and neuroendocrine support, with therapeutic doses of 15 to 45 mg per day, divided. While MK7 is excellent for cardiovascular and bone prevention, MK4 shows superior potency in specific treatments, especially when we are seeking deep genomic action.

Omega-3, EPA and DHA, is considered fuel for the brain and a natural anti-inflammatory. These are essential fatty acids found in cold-water fish, with anti-inflammatory, neuroprotective, and cardiovascular properties. It helps cognitive function, memory, mood, lowers triglycerides, and helps treat chronic inflammation. It is always important to verify purity, origin, free of heavy metals, and the balance between EPA and DHA. Ideally, they should be stored in amber-colored packaging so they do not oxidize with light exposure. There are many cheap brands on the market that do not provide the appropriate benefits, so seek recommendations for a quality omega-3 validated by your doctor. Yes, omega-3 is one of the most romanticized, consumed, and studied supplements, but its use requires extra attention precisely because of the unstable nature of polyunsaturated fats, PUFAs, such as EPA and DHA. These molecules are highly susceptible to oxidation by heat, light, and oxygen, a phenomenon that can occur from the moment the fish is caught until the supplement is bottled. What I mean is that if the fisherman exposes your deep cold-water fish to the heat of land, you will not get quality omega extraction, but rather a product that has lost its anti-inflammatory properties and starts generating free radicals and toxic products, such as lipid aldehydes, which can damage cell membranes and mitochondria. Even encapsulated supplements in dark bottles with purity certificates do not guarantee the absence of oxidation if there is no refrigerated production chain, controlled atmosphere, and the addition of antioxidants such as tocopherols.

Considered the guardian of immunity and cellular regeneration, zinc participates in DNA synthesis, tissue regeneration, and hormone production. It is essential for the immune system and for male fertility. It also helps fight acne, supports healing, and promotes mental health. It is worth noting that prolonged use requires monitoring or association with copper to avoid imbalances.

Selenium is a powerful antioxidant, necessary for thyroid gland function and for defense against free radicals. It helps immunity, the thyroid, cancer prevention, and cellular protection. The dose must be controlled, because excess is toxic. Foods such as Brazil nuts already provide a good amount, and two units a day can make a difference and help you.

In addition, selenium is an antidote to mercury poisoning. Mercury exhibits much of its toxicity by displacing selenium in key enzymes, but by adding extra selenium, one sees increased mercury excretion, reduced oxidative damage, and reduced toxicity. In other words, selenium supplementation binds to mercury and helps eliminate it, while also preventing oxidative stress. If you received vaccines that contain the preservative thimerosal, mercury, take selenium.

We also have iron, which is essential but should always be used with caution. It is fundamental for oxygen transport in the blood and for cognitive functions. Iron deficiency can cause anemia, fatigue, and hair loss. It is indicated for pregnant women and in cases of low ferritin. It should always be monitored through testing. Excess is pro-oxidant and inflammatory. One should avoid taking it with calcium and prefer to take it with vitamin C.

With the goal of rebalancing the foundation of your health, your gut, we have probiotics, which are beneficial microorganisms that restore the balance of the intestinal microbiota, directly impacting immunity, mood, and digestion. They are indicated in cases of dysbiosis, after antibiotics, intestinal disorders, allergies, and even depression. But pay attention, it is necessary to choose the right formula for the desired objective and rotate strains periodically.

Many health benefits are attributed to vitamin A. It is essential for the production of all steroid hormones, and it has already been shown to be superior to steroids themselves in the masculinization process. In one study, boys who received 6,000 IU per day of vitamin A showed improved height, among other benefits.

Another relevant point is this vitamin's relationship with wrinkle prevention, since collagen production and degradation are processes regulated by vitamin A. During supplementation, an improvement in skin aging is observed. Studies with up to 200,000 IU per day of retinol have demonstrated remission of severe acne and intestinal inflammation, lowering elevated serotonin.

Poor vision is one of the most common signs of vitamin A deficiency. It is important to highlight that zinc is necessary for all aspects of vitamin A metabolism, so an apparent deficiency of this vitamin may, in fact, be due to a lack of zinc. In addition, it is fundamental to maintain adequate levels of vitamin D to prevent vitamin A toxicity, and the reverse is also true.

B-complex vitamins are essential for providing energy and helping the central nervous system function harmoniously. It is a set of essential vitamins for energy metabolism, neurotransmitter formation, skin, nails, and brain function. It helps combat stress, mental fatigue, PMS, and neurological health. For example, vitamin B6 deficiency is related to symptoms such as unexplained itching, neurodermatitis and eczema, histamine intolerance, anxiety, insomnia, joint pain, and difficulty metabolizing proteins. This happens because B6 is a fundamental cofactor for enzymes that degrade histamine, such as DAO, convert sulfur, to form glutathione and sulfate, and reduce oxalate production. Before supplementing B-complex vitamins, it is essential to perform a biochemical assessment, evaluate the methylation cycle, and assess microbiota status. It is worth remembering that excessive supplementation can lead to neuropathy.

Vitamin C is the classic one for immunity and collagen. It is a potent antioxidant and cofactor for collagen production, immunity, and iron absorption. It helps prevent colds and flu, improves healing, and protects the skin and blood vessels. It is water-soluble, and the excess is eliminated in urine. Very high doses can cause intestinal discomfort, and splitting the dose may be more efficient.

We also have curcumin and quercetin, intelligent antioxidants, but they should be administered in rotation. Both are natural substances with anti-inflammatory, antiviral, and cell-protective action. Curcumin comes from turmeric, and quercetin is present in apples, onions, and colorful vegetables. They help modulate the immune system, protect the brain, reduce silent inflammation, and help prevent chronic diseases. They should be used in short cycles, for example, 3 months of use, alternating with other substances. Continuous use of antioxidants may impair natural cellular signaling.

One of the supplements currently being studied, and which, when used correctly, brings many benefits, is creatine, widely used by athletes, but known to go far beyond the sports universe.

For a long time seen only as a supplement for bodybuilders, creatine now occupies a prominent place in functional medicine, neurology, and even the health of aging. It is a compound naturally produced by the body, from amino acids such as arginine, glycine, and methionine, stored mainly in muscles and, to a lesser degree, in the brain and other tissues.

Its main function is to provide rapid energy for cells, especially in the form of phosphocreatine, which helps regenerate ATP, the body's energy currency. But its benefits go far beyond muscle strength.

In addition to increasing strength and muscle mass, it improves physical performance and accelerates recovery. This is especially relevant for older adults, who suffer from the natural loss of muscle mass, sarcopenia. Studies show that creatine supplementation, even without intense exercise, can preserve lean mass, improve balance, and prevent falls.

Another benefit is that creatine may improve brain function by optimizing ATP supply, since the brain consumes an enormous amount of energy. Studies show that it improves memory, focus, logical reasoning, and cognitive performance, especially in situations of sleep deprivation, stress, or in vegetarians. In addition, there is promising research on the use of creatine as an adjunct in conditions such as depression, Parkinson's disease, and Alzheimer's disease, because of its neuronal-protective and antioxidant action. Rat studies have shown that inhaled creatine may be a strategy for increasing its serum levels in the brain, important for Alzheimer's disease. Intranasal administration may circumvent the blood-brain barrier and deliver medications directly to the brain.

Creatine also has positive impacts on bone metabolism, stimulating bone-forming cells, osteoblasts, and helping prevent osteopenia and osteoporosis. It may also improve insulin sensitivity and contribute to glycemic control.

It is important to demystify this: creatine is not a hormone, it is not an anabolic steroid, and it does not harm the kidneys in healthy people. On the contrary, it is a nutrient with therapeutic potential, accessible, safe, and with much broader applications than previously imagined.

Another supplement you should know is taurine, an amino acid essential for the body's proper functioning and one that has impressive benefits for health, energy, and longevity. Taurine lowers blood pressure and improves insulin resistance, combats oxidative stress and chronic inflammation, protects the brain by reducing neuroinflammation and increasing dopamine, improves insulin sensitivity, helping control blood sugar, increases mitochondrial function, favoring energy and physical performance, accelerates muscle recovery and reduces post-workout soreness, supports cardiovascular health by lowering the risk of heart disease, regulates the immune system, helping fight infections, and improves sleep quality by reducing anxiety and improving relaxation. Important: do not take it on your own. Seek a healthcare professional to guide you.

Glycine is an amino acid that is special to me. At such a low cost, it literally has the power to prolong life, interrupt inflammation, heal your gut, and provide deep, restorative sleep. It is essential for various functions in the body and a powerful ally for those seeking health and well-being. It plays a fundamental role in protein synthesis, strengthening the immune system, joint health, and brain function. In addition, studies show that glycine may help with deep, restorative sleep by acting as a calming neurotransmitter, helping reduce anxiety and promote relaxation. It is vital for detoxification, therapeutic for schizophrenia, prevents excessive urination and foamy urine, antiviral, among so many other benefits. It can be taken at night to enhance its effects on sleep. Glycine has a high safety profile, but it is always important to consult a healthcare professional for individualized guidance. I use 5 to 10 grams a day, and it has a spectacular effect on my intestinal health.

Among the many supplements that attract interest because of their systemic and multifunctional effects, N-acetylcysteine, or simply NAC, stands out as a true key piece in maintaining cellular health. Derived from the amino acid cysteine, this molecule is much more than a mere supplement. It is the precursor of one of the most powerful antioxidants in our body: glutathione.

Glutathione acts like a kind of internal shield, protecting cells against damage caused by oxidative stress, a silent process that is nevertheless deeply involved in aging and chronic diseases. And NAC, by providing the raw material for glutathione production, becomes a strategic agent for preserving the body's biochemical balance.

In recent years, it has gained prominence in neuroscience and psychiatry because of its glutamate-modulating role, the main excitatory neurotransmitter of the central nervous system. Excess glutamate is associated with a series of mental disorders, including treatment-resistant depression, obsessive-compulsive disorder, schizophrenia, and even addictive behaviors such as addiction to drugs, cigarettes, or food. NAC acts as a brake in this system, helping restore neurochemical balance in a subtle yet effective way. Randomized studies have shown that 2,400 to 3,000 mg per day of NAC can significantly reduce obsessive symptoms,

OCD, as well as symptoms of schizophrenia, Parkinson's disease, and treatment-resistant major depression.

In the context of metabolic health and longevity, NAC also proves to be an important ally. Its antioxidant role contributes to reducing chronic inflammation, improving insulin sensitivity, and supporting muscle recovery after intense exercise. Men with fertility difficulties, for example, may benefit from its action by improving sperm quality through the reduction of oxidative stress in the testicles.

Another important point is that the efficacy of NAC is even more robust when it acts together with other synergistic nutrients, such as vitamin C, selenium, and zinc, all crucial for the full functioning of the endogenous antioxidant system.

These supplements represent a top ten not only because of popularity, but because of their functional relevance in the body. I could talk about many others here. Even so, it is worth reinforcing that supplementing is not accumulating capsules. It is making conscious choices, with criteria, based on testing and professional guidance. The secret lies in balance, personalization, and the quality of each compound used.

In a world marked by nutrient-depleted diets, worn-out soils, constant exposure to pesticides, and an increasingly stressful lifestyle, supplementing has ceased to be a luxury and has become a strategic health necessity. The human body, although extraordinary in its capacity for adaptation, needs quality substrates to function well, regenerate, protect itself, and evolve.

Throughout this chapter, we have seen that supplementing does not mean filling the shelf with capsules, but rather treating real illnesses and correcting nutritional deficiencies with intelligence, individualization, and purpose. It means understanding that nutrients do not act in isolation, but in complex networks of synergies and antagonisms, where too much of one can block another, and where the lack of one link can compromise the entire chain. Therefore, I say again, do not supplement on your own. Seek a professional who can help you manage it correctly and bring benefits to your health.

Understanding bioactive forms, the interactions among vitamins and minerals, the body's cycles, and the importance of rotation is what distinguishes efficient use from potentially toxic use. Nor can we ignore the influence of genetic polymorphisms, which alter the way each body metabolizes and makes use of nutrients. Modern health demands personalization, laboratory assessment, and listening to the body.

More than simply improving immunity, energy, or cognitive performance, supplementation can be a tool for biological shielding, protecting fertility, favoring a healthy pregnancy, and even helping prevent neurobehavioral diseases in babies who have not even been born yet. This is preventive medicine in its essence.

We are living through a generation of infertility, neurodevelopmental disorders, autoimmune diseases, and chronic fatigue, often silent. And if we do not look at the foundation, which is cellular nutrition, we will continue trying to remedy problems without understanding the root. Enough with saying that supplementation is quackery and that we are throwing money away.

Therefore, supplementing consciously is more than a personal choice: it is an act of care for the present and of responsibility for the future. It is investing in yourself, in your family, and in a healthier, more fertile, more awake generation.

May this chapter serve as a starting point for a new way of looking at self-care, with less trend-chasing and more knowledge, with less excess and more discernment, with less fear and more connection with one's own body.

Task:

- Take inventory of the supplements you use and research the quality and bioavailability of each one.

____
____
____
____

- Choose two essential supplements for your routine and begin monitoring their effects.

____
____
____
____

CHAPTER 4

INTERMITTENT FASTING AND CALORIC RESTRICTION

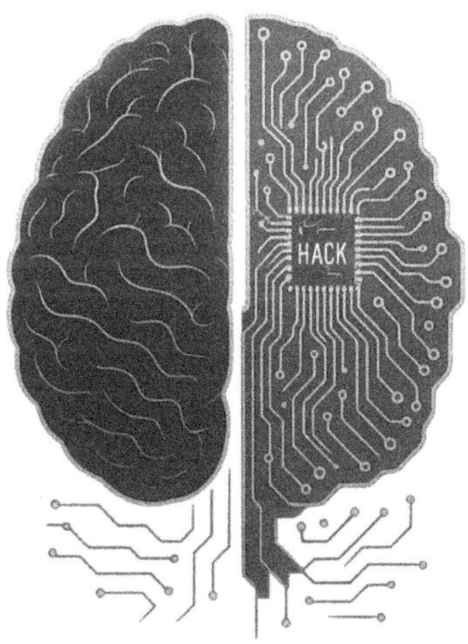

Intermittent fasting has become increasingly popular because of its potential health benefits, such as weight loss, improved metabolic health, and increased longevity. The concept of fasting is simple: it consists of periods of eating followed by periods of abstaining from food, varying in duration and frequency.

In the context of fasting, it is important to understand the distinctions between caloric fasting and metabolic fasting. Caloric fasting refers to the restriction of calories consumed over a period of time. In metabolic fasting, you may consume far fewer calories, or even none, during the fasting period, which forces the body to use its energy reserves, generally in the form of fat, to sustain its functions.

Metabolic fasting is related to the physiological changes that occur in the body in response to fasting. During this process, the body enters a fat-burning state and begins to produce ketone bodies, a source of energy derived from fatty acids. Fasting does not involve only the restriction of macronutrients, proteins, carbohydrates, and fats, but also the preservation and optimization of micronutrients, vitamins and minerals, essential for the body's proper functioning.

A fundamental aspect of fasting is the preservation of healthy fats, which continue to be a source of energy during the fasting period and contribute to proper brain function and cellular health.

To understand the main differences a little better:

Characteristic	**Caloric Fasting**	**Metabolic Fasting**
Caloric Fasting	Does not consume any	May use fats, such as coconut oil, ghee butter, olive oil, and MCT
Main objective	Total caloric restriction	Keep the body in a fat-burning state or ketosis
Permitted example	Only water, coffee, and tea without sweetener	Coffee with coconut oil or ghee, bone broth

Studies show that intermittent fasting and caloric restriction have been shown to influence several cellular processes, with significant impacts on health and longevity.

Fasting is a true reset for the body, promoting cellular cleanup, regeneration, and protection against various diseases. Depending on the duration and type of fasting, the effects may be more intense. One of the main mechanisms activated during fasting is autophagy.

Autophagy is a process of cellular cleanup in which the body destroys and recycles damaged or dysfunctional cellular components. This mechanism is crucial for maintaining cellular health, preventing the accumulation of damaged proteins, and reducing the risk of various diseases, including neurodegenerative diseases such as Alzheimer's and Parkinson's.

During fasting, autophagy is activated because of the lack of nutrients, forcing cells to optimize their resources and remove damaged parts. This process not only improves cellular health, but also has implications for longevity, since efficient cellular recovery can increase the body's resistance to stress and delay cellular aging.

Fasting is also associated with reduced risk of chronic diseases such as type 2 diabetes, cardiovascular disease, and cancer. Intermittent fasting and caloric restriction improve insulin sensitivity, reduce inflammation, and help control glucose and fat metabolism. This reduces the risk of insulin resistance and other risk factors for chronic diseases.

Research suggests that by improving metabolic efficiency and promoting cellular regeneration through autophagy, fasting may prolong lifespan and promote more robust health. In fasting, we have a great ally for integral health.

But how do you practice intermittent fasting?

There are several intermittent fasting protocols, each with its own characteristics and adaptations according to the individual's needs. The choice of the ideal protocol depends on each person's metabolism, goals, and daily routine.

I want to highlight the most common types of intermittent fasting protocols:

- 16/8 fasting: This consists of fasting for 16 hours and eating during an 8-hour window, done twice a week. This is one of the most popular protocols and can be adapted easily for most people. It would mean having your last meal of the day at 7:00 p.m. and the next day's meal at 1:00 p.m.
- 5:2 fasting: In this protocol, the person eats normally for five days of the week and restricts calories, approximately 500 to 600 calories, on the other two non-consecutive days. It is important to space these two calo-

rie-restriction days throughout the week, avoiding doing them back to back, for example, Monday and Thursday.

- 24-hour fasting: This involves fasting for 24 hours, in my recommendation once a week, and I prefer Monday. During this period, the body enters a deeper state of ketosis and autophagy.

The choice of protocol should take into account factors such as level of physical activity, body composition, and the ability to tolerate longer periods without food. For individuals with a higher level of physical activity, a more flexible protocol may be necessary, or periods of food intake focused on proteins and micronutrients may need to be included to avoid loss of muscle mass.

It is also essential to listen to your own body. Some people may feel fine with longer fasting, while others may need shorter windows. In clinical practice, if you feel hungry, have a headache, or feel tired, drink water with salt, it is probably just dehydration. If you notice you are going too far and feel unsafe, break the fast with fruit, so you will have a quick and nourishing source of glucose.

Although intermittent fasting has many benefits, it can also cause side effects that may vary from person to person, but the most common include intense hunger, fatigue, dizziness, headache, irritability, and constipation. For this reason, I advise you to seek specialized guidance before starting, and begin gradually.

Intermittent fasting has stopped being a passing trend and has established itself as a powerful tool for metabolic health, longevity, and mental clarity. However, in order to reap its benefits safely and sustainably, it is essential to understand its mechanisms, respect the body's signals, and follow a conscious, individualized approach.

During fasting, the body enters a state of detoxification and energy adaptation. In this process, there is a natural loss of fluids and electrolytes, which can lead to symptoms such as headache, fatigue, and dizziness. For that reason, staying well hydrated is essential. Plain water, unsweetened teas, and even black coffee, in moderation, help maintain energy and reduce appetite. Adding natural salt to water or using electrolytes can prevent drops in sodium, potassium, and magnesium, three minerals essential for cellular balance.

The end of a fast is just as important as the fast itself. Avoiding spikes in insulin and glucose is essential to preserve the metabolic benefits achieved. For that reason, meals with good nutrient density, rich in protein, healthy fats, and fiber, such as eggs, avocado, vegetables, and olive oil, help maintain satiety and stabilize metabolism. Avoiding ultra-processed foods and simple sugars is essential so as not to sabotage the positive effects of fasting.

When we fast, we lose more than just calories. Important minerals are also eliminated through urine. Deficiency in sodium, magnesium, and potassium can impair physical and mental performance. For that reason, foods such as leafy greens, avocado, nuts, and the strategic supplementation of electrolytes during the eating window can make all the difference for well-being.

For those who have never practiced fasting, the ideal is to start slowly. Beginning with 12 hours and gradually moving to 14 or 16 hours helps the body adapt without generating metabolic stress. Biological individuality must always be respected, there is no perfect fast, only the one that works in a balanced way for each person.

Many people ask whether it is safe to train while fasting. The answer is: it depends on the type of exercise, the intensity, and the level of metabolic adaptation. Light and moderate workouts are generally well tolerated, while high-intensity exercise may be more appropriate during the eating window. A black coffee before training can provide an extra boost without breaking the fast.

Little by little, just as I am adapted to fasting workouts, including long-distance runs of 18 km or lasting around 1 hour and 40 minutes, you will be too.

It is worth saying that fasting and self-care go hand in hand. Sleeping poorly or living under chronic stress can disrupt hunger hormones, such as ghrelin and leptin, and make fasting more difficult. Breathing techniques, meditation, yoga, and good sleep hygiene are essential for balancing cortisol and keeping the nervous system regulated. Fasting cannot be a poorly managed tool in the middle of a toxic and disorganized lifestyle. It is good to remember that many people reading this book skip meals, do not organize their day, do not practice morning rituals, or even basic sleep hygiene. The truth is that in the globalized world, we chase money, eat fast food, and skip meals, forcing a fast that, besides intensifying stress, will bring, at the end of the day, ravenous hunger, binge eating, lack of control, and obesity.

One of the most impressive effects of fasting lies in the way it changes the brain's energy source. When glucose stores are low, the liver converts fatty acids into ketone bodies, which become the body's new fuel. This not only promotes body fat burning, but also improves focus, mental clarity, and energy.

The three main ketone bodies are:

- Acetoacetate, AcAc: the first produced by the liver.
- Beta-hydroxybutyrate, BHB: the most efficient one, used mainly by the brain and muscles. It can be supplemented during fasting, and 3 grams will increase metabolic activity, with that, the production of ketone bodies through fat burning and consequently greater weight loss.
- Acetone: a byproduct eliminated through the breath and urine, responsible for ketone breath.

Studies show that BHB has neuroprotective, anti-inflammatory, and even gene-modulating actions related to longevity. It improves neuronal plasticity and reduces oxidative stress in the brain, which is one of the explanations for the improved focus and cognitive performance in people who practice fasting regularly.

By understanding the role of ketone bodies, the importance of nutrition during the eating window, and the signals the body gives, fasting stops being a fad and becomes a lasting ally in the pursuit of health, focus, and vitality.

Urine tests, reagent strips measure acetoacetate, blood tests, which measure beta-hydroxybutyrate, and breath tests, which detect acetone, are the indicators used to know whether we are producing ketone bodies.

And when that happens, we will have several benefits such as improved focus and mental clarity, fat burning, reduced blood sugar spikes, and a neuroprotective effect. Studies indicate several benefits for diseases such as Alzheimer's and epilepsy. Our patients at the Melo Institute of Integrative Medicine use ketone body evaluation strips, just as diabetics use strips to evaluate glucose, for fasting control and monitoring weight loss.

More than simply not eating, fasting is a way to give the digestive system a pause and rest, improve insulin sensitivity, modulate inflammation, and promote autophagy, a natural process of cellular cleanup. It is an ancestral practice, backed by modern science, that can promote more energy, lightness, and mental clarity when done intelligently.

Intermittent fasting is a powerful tool, provided that it is applied with awareness, knowledge, and listening to one's own body. It is not a competition to see who can fast the longest, nor a form of dietary punishment. It is a choice of self-care, in which the quality of food, adequate hydration, rest, and emotional balance are just as important as the time spent without eating.

It is worth emphasizing that some people may experience difficulty at the beginning of the practice of fasting. In order to improve cognitive performance during fasting, it is important to:

Avoid excessive consumption of coffee and other stimulating beverages, which may cause energy spikes followed by crashes.

Ensure high-quality nutrition during eating windows, with nutrients essential for the brain, such as essential fatty acids, omega-3, B-complex vitamins, and antioxidants.

Practice stress-management techniques, such as meditation and deep breathing, to help maintain mental clarity during periods without food.

Intermittent fasting and caloric restriction offer powerful health benefits, including the activation of autophagy, increased longevity, and reduced risk of chronic diseases. However, adapting to these practices should be done carefully and with awareness of your metabolism, preferences, and nutritional needs.

I believe that with the right approach and proper adjustment of the fasting protocol, it is possible to avoid side effects, optimize cognitive performance, and improve overall health in the long term.

And now that you have learned about intermittent fasting, shall we put it into practice? I want to leave you with a few suggestions:

1. Start slowly. Try a 12-to-14-hour fasting protocol and record how you feel.
2. If you already fast, begin varying the times or adding days of prolonged fasting.

CHAPTER 5

PHYSICAL ACTIVITY AND PERFORMANCE

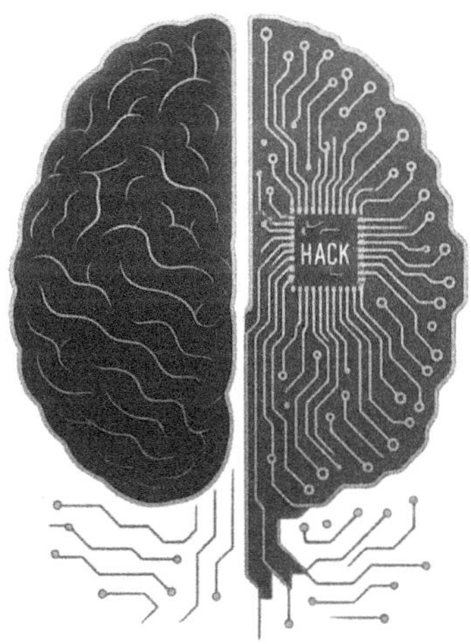

The relationship between physical activity and performance has been the subject of study and interest throughout history, from the athletes of Ancient Greece to the high-performance competitors of today. The pursuit of better performance, whether in elite sports or in day-to-day activities, involves a complex interaction among physiological, psychological, and environmental factors.

In this chapter, I will explore how regular exercise can impact physical and mental capacity, analyzing the main components that influence performance, such as strength, endurance, flexibility, and recovery. I will also address evidence-based strategies to optimize performance, considering aspects such as nutrition, rest, and training planning.

Understanding the mechanisms behind physical activity and its influence on human performance is not relevant only for athletes and coaches, but also for anyone who wants to improve health and quality of life through movement.

Certainly, you have already heard or been advised to exercise, or you already exercise in some way. So I ask: what importance does physical activity have in your life? What do you think about it? Stop for a moment and reflect on that. I remember perfectly how I felt in medical school, and what awakened me to the practice of physical activity. It was in 2008. I did not usually take the bus, but sometimes I needed to run to college because I had overslept. During those runs, I felt chest pain because of my complete lack of physical conditioning. I was not any superhuman, much less a biohacker, I was just a skinny kid who smoked hand-rolled cigarettes, drank at the college bar, and had no set bedtime.

That was how I gradually realized I was sabotaging my own health. It took me two semesters to accept it. I lived tired and discouraged, and I was never good at sports. The truth really hit me when I had to retake cardiology. That made me reflect. From then on, I began, day after day, to move away from my old habits and get closer to the gym. And then I became "that annoying guy." I started thinking about health all the time. I became the unbearable one in the student house, the one everyone avoided when the subject was going out, drinking beer, or eating pizza late at night. In fact, I had a few arguments with my housemates.

Regular physical activity has a significant impact on longevity and quality of life. Different types of training, such as strength training, HIIT, High-Intensity Interval Training, and aerobic training, offer distinct but equally powerful benefits for the human body.

Strength training, especially resistance training, is one of the most effective ways to combat aging because it helps preserve muscle mass, which is crucial as we grow older. The loss of muscle mass is related to a series of health problems, such as bone fragility and increased risk of falls, in addition to reducing basal metabolism.

Basal metabolism is the amount of energy the body needs to maintain vital functions at rest. It is the energy required for the body to function without performing any physical activity.

Maintaining muscular strength through strength training not only improves mobility and functional independence, but may also increase longevity. Studies show that people who engage in regular strength training tend to have a lower risk of chronic diseases, such as type 2 diabetes and cardiovascular disease.

HIIT, High-Intensity Interval Training, is a training strategy that combines high-intensity exercise with short rest periods.

This type of workout has been widely studied because of its positive impact on cardiovascular health, insulin sensitivity, and body composition. It is highly time-efficient, providing significant benefits in shorter sessions.

The impact of HIIT on longevity is related to its ability to improve mitochondrial function and increase the efficiency of the cardiovascular system. HIIT also activates the anaerobic metabolic pathway, which allows for more efficient fat burning and improved metabolic health, both essential for slowing aging.

Aerobic training, such as running, cycling, or swimming, improves cardiovascular system health, increasing lung capacity and improving blood circulation, factors directly linked to longevity. In addition, aerobic exercise has positive effects on body weight, blood pressure control, and the reduction of bad cholesterol, LDL.

Regular aerobic activity also promotes the production of endorphins, contributing to mental and emotional health, in addition to helping reduce the risk of chronic diseases such as hypertension, type 2 diabetes, and even certain types of cancer.

Maximizing mitochondrial production and optimizing VO2 max are fundamental goals for athletes and individuals seeking to improve endurance and aerobic performance. The mitochondrion is the cell's "power plant," responsible for ATP, adenosine triphosphate, production through cellular respiration. The greater the mitochondrial density, the greater the body's capacity to generate energy efficiently.

VO_2 max, in turn, represents the maximum oxygen consumption during intense exercise and is one of the best indicators of aerobic fitness. It depends on factors such as the heart's ability to pump blood, the efficiency of gas exchange in the lungs, and muscle capillarization.

The combination of specific training, proper nutrition, and recovery strategies can stimulate mitochondrial biogenesis and optimize VO_2 max. Methods such as High-Intensity Interval Training, continuous aerobic training, exposure to hypoxia, and strategic supplementation, for example creatine, nitrates, and polyphenols, are some of the approaches used to achieve these goals. VO_2 max, maximum oxygen consumption, is one of the most powerful predictors of longevity. If you train with the goal of increasing your VO2 max, you are on the right path and will probably be long-lived. A robust scientific study on this was published in JAMA, Journal of the American Medical Association, in 2018. It evaluated more than 122,000 participants and demonstrated a strong inverse association between VO_2 max and all-cause mortality. Physical fitness was more predictive of mortality than smoking, hypertension, type 2 diabetes, and coronary disease. Maintaining or improving VO_2 max with regular aerobic training, such as running, cycling, swimming, or HIIT, may be one of the most effective strategies for living longer and with better quality of life.

Although traditional aerobic exercise is still the foundation, especially high-intensity interval training, HIIT, and zone 2 endurance, as Peter Attia teaches us in his book Outlive (2023), modern science and biohacking offer technologies capable of amplifying or even simulating these effects.

One of them is hypoxia masks, which simulate high altitudes by reducing the concentration of inhaled oxygen. This forces the body to adapt, increasing the production of red blood cells and the efficiency of oxygen uptake, which directly improves VO_2 max. Even more effective is intermittent hypoxic training, IHT, which alternates short periods of rarefied air with normal breathing, stimulating EPO production, angiogenesis, and greater mitochondrial density, even at rest. But take it easy, do not do anything without a professional. Following the same logic, there is the "live high, train low" strategy, in which one sleeps in low-oxygen environments, using hypoxia tents, and trains at sea level, like our Brazilian triathlete Thiago Vinhal. This allows the hematological benefits of altitude without compromising training intensity. Another interesting alternative is the use of blood flow restriction bands, BFR, which produce cardiovascular and muscular adaptations with light loads, ideal for those seeking time efficiency or who have joint limitations. I love blood flow restriction and use it almost daily. My device is the Kaatsu, modern, practical, safe, and accessible.

Heat is also an ally. Frequent sauna exposure, for example, increases plasma volume and improves endothelial function, simulating the effects of aerobic training at rest. In addition, photobiomodulation with red and infrared light stimulates mitochondrial activity, optimizing the use of oxygen by the cells. Although it does not replace exercise, this technology enhances gains, especially when applied before training. Finally, mitochondrial supplementation comes in as support. Compounds such as CoQ10, PQQ, L-carnitine, creatine, nitrate-rich beets, and NAD^+ precursors, such as NMN or NR, improve mitochondrial function and cellular aerobic capacity. When combined, these resources strategically expand physiological limits, accessing the maximum potential of performance and longevity, even for those who cannot train like an athlete.

Moving on, physical training plays a crucial role in mitochondrial biogenesis, the process by which cells increase the number of mitochondria. Exercises that demand high intensity, such as HIIT and aerobic training, are especially effective in this process. These types of training increase the number of mitochondria in muscle cells and promote significant improvements in physical performance.

In addition, resistance training, such as strength training, also helps improve mitochondrial function, especially in slow-twitch muscles, type 1, which depend more heavily on mitochondria for energy production. This contributes to greater endurance and muscle recovery.

VO2 max is one of the best indicators of a person's aerobic capacity. It represents the maximum amount of oxygen a person can consume during high-intensity exercise. Improving VO2 max is directly related to improving cardiovascular efficiency and the body's ability to use oxygen more effectively.

As said before, to optimize VO2 max, it is essential to perform regular high-intensity aerobic exercise, such as fast running or intense cycling, and to practice exercises that challenge the cardiovascular system, such as HIIT. The combination of proper training intensity and volume can increase the capacity to consume and use oxygen, which improves performance and overall endurance.

Let us go back to heart rate zone 2. Zone 2 is an exercise intensity range in which the heart beats at a moderate rate, usually between 60 to 70% of maximum heart rate. Training in this zone is highly effective for fat burning and improving aerobic capacity without causing major stress to the body. Among its various benefits, these are worth highlighting:

Fat burning: during zone 2 training, the body uses mainly fat as its energy source, which helps reduce body fat over time.

Improved aerobic capacity, because exercises in zone 2 increase the efficiency of the cardiovascular and respiratory systems, promoting long-term improvement in cardiovascular health.

Zone 2 training is ideal for those who want to improve endurance without overloading the joints or muscular system. In addition, it allows longer training sessions without causing a high level of fatigue.

Training in zone 2 can also be useful as a foundation for other, more intense types of training, helping the body adapt and improving overall performance because it does not present danger for most healthy people. On the contrary, this type of training is highly beneficial for cardiovascular health, aerobic endurance, and mitochondrial efficiency.

Possible risks and considerations that I need to highlight, and you need to pay attention to:

- If there is an excessive increase in training load without adequate recovery, chronic fatigue or even overtraining may occur.
- People with heart problems should always consult a doctor before starting any aerobic exercise program.
- Dehydration and electrolyte imbalances: even at moderate intensities, long training periods may lead to loss of fluids and essential minerals.

When done correctly, zone 2 training is safe and extremely effective for improving aerobic endurance and mitochondrial function.

Strategies for Accelerated Recovery and Reduction of Oxidative Stress

Recovery is an essential aspect of improving performance and preventing injuries, especially after intense training. Reducing oxidative stress and optimizing recovery processes are fundamental for maintaining good physical and mental health.

There are several strategies for effective accelerated recovery:

- Quality Sleep: sleep is fundamental for muscle recovery and cellular regeneration. During deep sleep, the body carries out many repair processes, including muscle protein synthesis and hormonal regulation. Later in this book, we will have a chapter on sleep.
- Post-Workout Nutrition: consuming a meal rich in proteins and carbohydrates after training helps replenish glycogen stores and repair muscles. Essential amino acids and antioxidants present in foods such as berries and green vegetables can accelerate recovery.
- Stretching and Mobility: incorporating stretching sessions and mobility exercises helps improve flexibility and reduce muscular stiffness, in addition to making pains previously unknown disappear.
- Active Recovery Techniques: light exercises, such as walking or easy-paced swimming, can help accelerate recovery and reduce the buildup of lactic acid.

Oxidative stress occurs when there is an imbalance between the production of free radicals and the body's ability to neutralize them. Strategies to reduce oxidative stress include:

- Natural Antioxidants: consuming foods rich in vitamins C and E, such as citrus fruits, nuts, and seeds, can help neutralize free radicals.
- Controlled Training: excessive training may increase oxidative stress. It is important to balance intense training with adequate rest periods.

In addition, techniques such as deep breathing and stretching can also reduce the effects of oxidative stress and improve muscle recovery.

Regular physical activity, including strength training, HIIT, and aerobic training, offers powerful benefits for health and longevity. Maximizing mitochondrial production, optimizing VO2 max, and training efficiently in heart rate zone 2 are key strategies for improving athletic performance and overall health.

However, it is important to remember that recovery and the reduction of oxidative stress play a fundamental role in the success of any training program. By adopting a balanced approach among exercise, nutrition, rest, and recovery, it is possible to achieve improved physical performance and ensure a healthier and longer life. Remember that information, knowledge, and proper guidance will make a difference.

So why not begin?

- Add 5 extra minutes of physical activity each day, it can be HIIT, strength training, or walking.
- Try a new type of exercise, such as sprinting, functional training, or mobility work.

CHAPTER 6

INFRARED LIGHT EXPOSURE

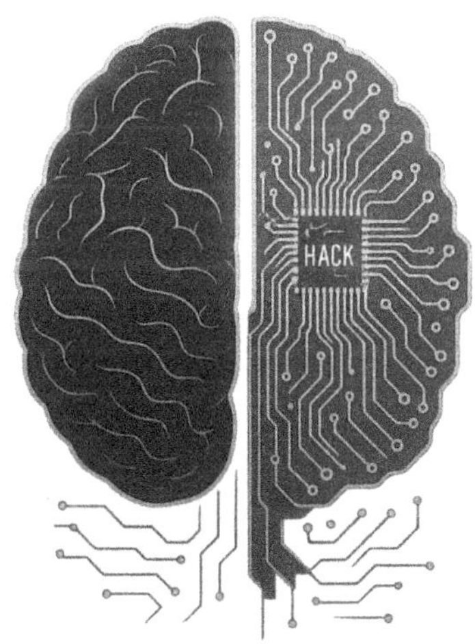

The discovery of red light therapy was actually an accident. In 1967, the Hungarian physician Endre Mester was trying to use lasers to treat tumors in rats. The lasers did not affect the tumors, but he observed something unexpected. As with several discoveries in medicine that happened by accident, do not judge something new, do not be the skeptic who points fingers and insults others by calling them denialists.

Going back to Dr. Endre, the areas treated with lasers showed accelerated hair growth and faster healing. This fortunate discovery changed everything.

How does light influence metabolism, cellular repair, and energy production, ATP?

Light, especially red and infrared wavelengths, can have a profound impact on many cellular and metabolic processes, mainly by interacting with mitochondria, water, collagen, oxygen, and various proteins. This happens because that light communicates with photosensors in the cells, activating various biochemical pathways, including those responsible for energy production and cellular repair.

Infrared light is a form of light that makes up about 50% of sunlight. It is also found in red light therapy devices, where its wavelengths range from approximately 700 nm to 3000 nm, further classified as near infrared, mid-infrared, and far infrared.

In medical and therapeutic practice, for those of you who want to know what device to buy and which wavelengths are the most studied, here is a tip. The two wavelengths most commonly used are 660 nm, which has more superficial penetration, and 850 nm, nearly invisible to the human eye, which can penetrate up to 40 mm. Generally, good devices feature both wavelengths, and their actions are synergistic.

660 nm, visible red light

- Range: visible red light
- Penetration: about 5 to 10 mm, skin and superficial tissues
- Main actions
- Stimulates collagen production;
- Accelerates wound healing;
- Reduces wrinkles and signs of aging;
- Treats acne and skin inflammation;
- Activates mitochondria in epithelial tissues.
- 850 nm, near infrared, NIR
- Range: near infrared, almost invisible to the human eye
- Penetration: 20 to 40 mm, muscles, joints, deep tissues
- Main actions
- Increases mitochondrial ATP
- Reduces muscle and joint pain;
- Improves circulation and tissue oxygenation;
- Supports recovery from muscle injuries;
- Modulates inflammatory processes.

These devices, which may be used secondarily, do not replace what sunlight naturally provides, and that is important to emphasize. They are especially useful if you live in cold places, areas with low sun exposure, or harsh winters, such as northern Canada, Alaska, Greenland, Norway, nearby regions, or even Chile. They are also recommended if you spend most of the day indoors with little or no exposure to natural light, such as in offices, hospitals, or factories. In addition, they may benefit older adults with limited mobility, people with chronic or autoimmune diseases, athletes in rehabilitation, and even individuals who suffer from seasonal depression. In these situations, daily infrared light therapy can be a very valuable complementary strategy.

When red and infrared light penetrate the skin, they are absorbed by the mitochondria in the cells. These cellular organelles are responsible for producing ATP, adenosine triphosphate, an organic molecule that stores energy in the cells of all living organisms. It is known as the cell's "energy currency." Light stimulates the mitochondria to produce more ATP, which can improve cellular metabolism, increase overall energy, and even improve metabolic efficiency.

ATP production is essential for processes such as muscle contraction, protein synthesis, and the maintenance of cellular functions. With more energy available, cells can function more efficiently, promoting better overall health.

Red and infrared light also play an important role in cellular repair. They can stimulate collagen synthesis and improve blood circulation in the treated area, speeding up recovery after injury and inflammation. Light can also increase the activation of growth factors, such as insulin-like growth factor, IGF-1, which plays a fundamental role in cellular repair and tissue regeneration.

In addition, studies suggest that red light can help reduce inflammation and relieve pain by modulating inflammatory mediators and neurotransmitters. This makes it useful in the treatment of muscle injuries, sprains, joint diseases, and even chronic pain conditions.

Red and infrared light are widely used in aesthetic therapies to improve skin health, treating everything from aging to acne and other inflammatory conditions. They promote collagen stimulation because red light penetrates the skin, stimulating the production of collagen and elastin, proteins essential for skin firmness and elasticity. This can help reduce wrinkles and sagging and improve the skin's overall appearance. It is easy to find, on sites such as Amazon, specific infrared and LED therapy technologies for facial treatments in the beauty care or health and wellness categories, such as facial masks for treating conditions and even facial rejuvenation.

Light therapy can help reduce inflammation, promoting recovery from skin conditions such as acne, rosacea, psoriasis, melasma, and others. Whether associated or not with vitamin C creams, collagen peptides, hyaluronic acid, and facial copper crystals, it can bring impressive benefits to the appearance and health of the skin.

The therapeutic use of infrared light can accelerate the healing of wounds such as cuts, burns, and scars by stimulating cellular regeneration and blood flow. This was one of the regular and daily treatments I used when, accidentally, a 75-inch TV came loose from a wall mount and, on impact, tore the tendon of the long head of my biceps. Without a doubt, daily infrared therapy, for about 10 to 15 minutes at the injury site, contributed to the healing, recovery, and restoration of the tendon after surgery.

These effects are obtained because of red light's ability to penetrate the dermal layer of the skin and influence blood circulation and the activity of not only superficial cells, but deeper ones as well.

Exposure to red light has also been shown to be effective in sleep regulation and improving the quality of rest, given that its use stimulates daytime and nighttime melatonin production.

Using red light before bed can help regulate circadian rhythm, which is the biological clock that controls sleep and wake cycles. At home, when I get back from work, I put on glasses to block blue light, turn off the Wi-Fi before going to sleep, and also try to do red light therapy associated with Pulsetto. That is certainly a biohacker lifestyle that makes a difference.

Red light, unlike blue light, such as that emitted by digital screens, does not interfere with the production of melatonin, the hormone that regulates sleep. This means it can be used to help with the transition to sleep without harming the quality of rest. By regulating circadian rhythm, red light can promote deeper, more restorative sleep, which is fundamental for immunity and healthy longevity.

Since mitochondria are essential for cellular energy production, mitochondrial health is fundamental to overall well-being. Red and infrared light therapies help improve mitochondrial function by stimulating mitochondria to produce more ATP and increase cellular energy efficiency.

Basically, infrared light is like fuel for your mitochondrial colony. We have to remember that the function of mitochondria goes far beyond bioenergetics; they influence a large part of our biology. That includes hormone synthesis. Yes, direct red light therapy on the scrotal sac can influence testosterone and sperm production in the testes through the mitochondrial pathway, just as directly on the scalp one can perform neurophotobiomodulation, influencing the mitochondrial activity of neurons. Mitochondria also act in heme production in blood cells, regulation and transcription of nuclear DNA and RNA through ROS signaling and biophotons, and, beyond that, via cellular organelles, immune responses, regulation of autophagy, and apoptosis.

Photobiomodulation, a process in which light is used to improve cellular function, is a therapy that has been explored to reduce mitochondrial aging, improve ATP production, and increase cellular resistance to stress. This has implications not only for daily energy, but also for muscle recovery, brain health, and even longevity.

However, when we are exposed to native electromagnetic fields, EMFs, sunlight, the geomagnetic field, Schumann resonance, and non-native EMFs, blue light, Wi-Fi, Bluetooth, microwaves, we have different responses in relation to health and toxicity. Chronic exposure to non-native EMFs dehydrates us. This happens through mitochondrial function, dysregulated calcium signaling, circadian disruption and aquaporin water channels*, inflammation, low redox level, and changes in hydrogen bonding in the water network, which supposedly are coupled to the electromagnetic field signals of Mother Nature. Electromagnetic pollution from pulsed electromagnetic fields, PEMFs, dysregulates our entire energy system, causing mitochondriopathy, but infrared therapy can positively influence self-regulation after exposure to PEMFs.

The quantum effects on water, through infrared light, have an absurd number of positive biological effects.

Here are some interesting ones:

- Charge separation in water occurs on all surfaces it touches, allowing a systemic flow of electrons, electricity, and protons, protonicity, permitting quantum communication of energy and information to the tissues that need it.
- The negative charge that coats our blood vessels, veins and arteries, assists in the efficient transfer of anything negatively charged within them, especially red blood cells, erythrocytes, which should have a strong negative charge on their outer layer. This is further enhanced by

grounding, which releases more electrons from Earth's net negative charge.

- This water also influences cerebrospinal fluid for the efficient transfer of neurotransmitters, hormones, and metabolites throughout the central nervous system, as well as the efficient removal of metabolic waste, debris, and toxins that are ejected into the lymphatic system, which is also greatly enhanced by this water in lymphatic vessels and nodes.
- Being quantum-coherent water, it is capable of using other biophysical and quantum effects, such as tunneling, entanglement, superposition, semiconduction, resonance and molecular vibrations, and much more.
- Addressing molecular resonances among various molecules, this is how we increase receptor sensitivity, DNA and RNA activity, cell membrane signaling, redox factors, and much more. That is certainly it. No. There is still more.
- Near-infrared light photons directly increase daytime melatonin production. This melatonin acts like a Swiss Army knife inside your body.

Here is just a small list of the action of daytime melatonin produced through infrared light:

- increases mitochondrial function, ATP, CO2, H2O;
- controls autophagy and apoptosis;
- upregulates endogenous antioxidant enzyme regulation, NRF2, SOD, CAT, GPX, TPX;
- upregulates glutathione and NADPH synthesis;

- has the capacity to recycle metabolites in our main redox cycle, vitamin C, vitamin E, glutathione, NADPH, etc.;
- acts as an antioxidant in its own right because of its electron-rich indole, including against hydroxyl radicals;
- influences various tissues and systems: liver, gut, kidneys, brain, immune system, muscles, sex organs, etc.;
- binds free heavy and transition metals for detoxification;
- modulates uncoupling proteins, UCP1, UCP2, UCP3;
- prevents intracellular calcium overload, $Ca2+$;
- controls photoreceptor regeneration;
- is easily transportable because of its fat-soluble and water-soluble properties;
- regulates aromatase activity, estrogen;

You may already be tired of so much theory. We already know that red light is an incredible biohacker therapy, but how can we incorporate red or infrared light into our daily lives? Incorporating it into your routine can be simple, depending on the devices you choose. Here are some practical ways to use light to benefit your health:

Use of Therapeutic Devices

1. Red Light and Infrared Lamps: Some red light therapeutic lamps or panels can be used at home. To take advantage of their benefits, you can apply the light directly to the desired area, for example, face, scalp, abdomen, testicles, muscles, or joints. Sessions of 10 to 20 minutes daily are common.

2. Red Light Masks: For those who want to improve skin health, red light masks are a great option. They can be used to treat acne, reduce fine lines, or simply improve the texture and appearance of the skin.

3. Light Therapy Beds or Devices: Some clinics offer treatments with infrared light beds or phototherapy devices that emit intense light to promote recovery and cellular rejuvenation.

Incorporating It Into Your Lifestyle

- Sun Exposure: During the day, a few minutes of sun exposure can also provide natural red and infrared light. Keeping direct contact with sunlight in the morning can help regulate circadian rhythms and improve melatonin production at night.
- Red Light Environments for Sleep: To improve sleep quality, consider installing soft red-light bulbs in your bedroom or using a red-light flashlight before bed to avoid blue light stimulation.

Although red and infrared light therapy is generally safe, it is important to avoid excessive exposure. Use light therapies according to the instructions to avoid adverse effects, such as eye discomfort or overheating. If you have any skin condition or specific health issue, it is important to consult a physician before starting any type of light therapy.

Red and infrared light offer significant health benefits, from promoting cellular repair and ATP production to improving skin health, sleep, and mitochondrial function.

Incorporating these therapies practically into your daily life can be an effective way to optimize your overall health and maximize the body's recovery and regeneration processes. With conscious and regular use, you can take advantage of their many benefits for a healthier and more balanced life.

Putting It Into Practice:

- Spend 10 minutes in the morning sun without dark sunglasses.
- If you have access to a red-light or infrared lamp, use it daily for 10 minutes and record how you feel.

* Aquaporin water, functional interpretation: This is an informal expression used by some integrative physicians and biohackers to refer to biologically active water, that is, water that is being correctly absorbed, directed, and used by the body through aquaporins.

CHAPTER 7

SAUNA AND HEAT THERAPY OR HYPERTHERMIA

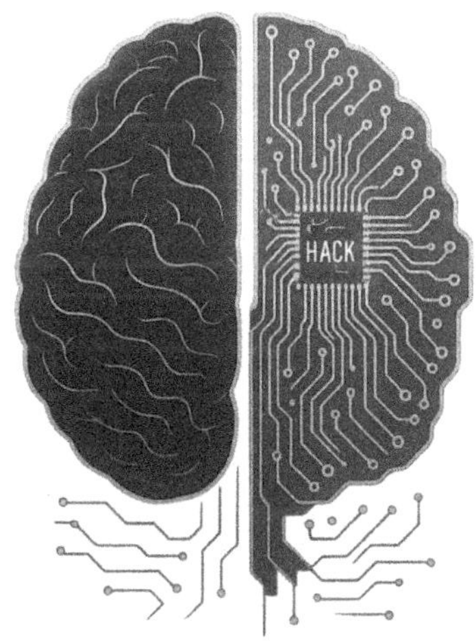

During the first wave of the COVID-19 pandemic, on March 29, 2020, when the world was still dominated by fear, misinformation, and the control of media narratives shaped by pharmaceutical interests, I treated a 37-year-old patient, Paula, who deeply trusted our physician-patient relationship.

At that moment, the benefits of corticosteroids in the treatment of COVID-19 were not yet known, since their use was established later. The turning point came with the publication of the preliminary results of the RECOVERY Trial on June 16, 2020, in the United Kingdom. This large randomized clinical trial demonstrated that dexamethasone, 6 mg per day for up to 10 days, significantly reduced mortality in hospitalized COVID-19 patients who required oxygen or mechanical ventilation when used in the second phase of the disease, known as the inflammatory phase.

The population was locked down, and the protocols were confusing and contradictory. However, I had already been closely following emerging clinical practices on the international scene, especially from hospitals in the New York region, which reported the safe and effective use of intravenous megadoses of vitamin C, between 40 and 70 grams, as an oxidizing and immunomodulatory tool.

I proposed to the patient an intervention that united scientific knowledge with integrative functional medicine: I laid her on the Biomat, a device made with amethyst stones that emits infrared pulses and heats up to 70 °C, and began a slow infusion of 20 grams of intravenous vitamin C. The patient wore a swimsuit and was wrapped in a blanket, over which we applied one of those thermal massage blankets, and we also heated the entire room with warm air, creating a true chamber of therapeutic heat, an improvised sauna for clinical purposes.

The goal of hyperthermia was to simulate a thermal response similar to fever, an essential physiological resource of the immune system, capable of increasing leukocyte motility, interferon efficiency, and NK cell activity, while at the same time inhibiting viral replication. Infrared heat, in turn, penetrates deeply into the tissues, promoting vasodilation, increased blood flow, and the release of nitric oxide, with the consequent improvement of tissue oxygenation. To enhance this oxygenation, I combined high-flow oxygen therapy, 7 L/min, inspired by von Ardenne therapy, and a 5 mg dose of tadalafil in order to amplify peripheral and pulmonary perfusion.

The patient, who arrived at the clinic with severe chest tightness, describing the sensation of carrying two bricks in her lungs, left the appointment a few hours later with surprising vigor, free from the pressure in her chest, with restored energy, and deeply impressed by the effectiveness of the treatment.

This experience was replicated with other COVID-19 patients, among them Walkiria, 62 years old, whom I had followed at the clinic since 2015. Her case illustrates how the intelligent use of therapeutic sauna, combined with the tools of functional medicine, can become a powerful early-intervention strategy in the face of viral respiratory infections.

Sauna and heat therapy, or hyperthermia, are practices that have gained considerable attention in recent years because of their benefits for health and longevity. Exposure to heat has profound effects on the body, stimulating a series of physiological responses that help improve cardiovascular health, promote detoxification, and even combat chronic disease.

In this context, the focus is on heat shock proteins, HSPs, which are proteins that help stabilize and transport intracellular proteins. They are found in all living organisms. They play an important role in maintaining cellular health, and in the way sauna can influence longevity, cardiovascular benefits, and even the fight against cancer. Let us explore these points in more detail.

When the body is exposed to heat, as in a sauna, it enters a state of thermal stress. This stress activates the production of heat shock proteins, HSPs, which are fundamental for cellular protection and recovery. HSPs play a crucial role in protection against cellular damage, including damage caused by oxidative stress, UV radiation, and toxins.

And how do HSPs work?

Heat shock proteins are molecules that help keep cells healthy under conditions of stress. They act in several ways, such as repairing damaged proteins. HSPs help correct damaged proteins that may occur during thermal stress. They also prevent protein aggregation, stopping damaged proteins from clumping together and forming structures that may be harmful to the cell. Another function is the promotion of autophagy. HSPs can stimulate the process of autophagy, a cellular mechanism that "cleans" the cell by removing damaged or dysfunctional components.

By promoting the expression of these proteins, sauna can help improve cellular resilience and slow the effects of aging. Over the long term, this may result in greater longevity, since cells become more efficient at repairing and protecting themselves against damage.

Studies suggest that regular exposure to heat, such as sauna use, may help delay cellular aging and reduce the incidence of age-related chronic diseases, such as heart disease, diabetes, and neurodegenerative diseases, through increased production of HSPs.

It is proven that sauna and heat therapy bring many cardiovascular benefits and promote detoxification of the body.

Sauna has a significant impact on heart health. When exposed to heat, the body reacts in a way similar to physical exercise, increasing heart rate and dilating blood vessels, which improves blood circulation and tissue oxygenation. This cardiovascular effect simulates the benefits of exercise without the need for intense physical effort.

There is an increase in heart rate, since during a sauna session, heart rate may rise from 60 to 70 beats per minute to 120 to 150 bpm, which increases blood flow and improves oxygen delivery to the tissues.

Exposure to heat also causes blood vessels to dilate, which may help reduce blood pressure and improve cardiovascular health. Studies show that sauna may help improve arterial elasticity, reducing the risk of cardiovascular disease.

In addition, sauna has been associated with a reduced risk of myocardial infarction, stroke, and premature death from heart disease. Regular practice may be an important strategy for improving cardiovascular health and reducing the risk of chronic disease.

Detoxification is another important benefit of sauna. Through heat-induced sweating, the body releases toxins, heavy metals, and other substances harmful to health. Although sauna does not replace a proper detoxification system, it can be a complementary tool to help eliminate toxins. Sweating helps release substances such as mercury, lead, and cadmium, which may accumulate in the body over time. It can also improve kidney function. By promoting the elimination of toxins through the skin, sauna may also reduce the workload on the kidneys and help eliminate metabolic waste.

It is known that sauna may also help reduce inflammation and improve the immune system, contributing to a better ability of the body to protect itself against disease.

I want to leave here my considerations regarding the dry sauna, the only technique I recommend and personally practice. The dry sauna, the traditional Finnish model, which is recognized worldwide for its health benefits and ancestral use, provides heat with low humidity, promoting a rapid elevation of skin temperature to around 40 °C in just a few minutes, while core body temperature rises only about 1 °C.

This thermal gradient diverts up to 70% of cardiac output to the skin, imitating the effects of moderate cardiovascular exercise without the need for physical movement. As a result, the heart pumps up to 70% more blood, something comparable to zone 3 aerobic training, directing 50 to 70% of blood flow to the skin, which favors vasodilation and improves peripheral circulation.

In addition, exposure to heat induces intense sweat production, between 0.6 and 1 kg per hour, facilitating detoxification through the skin. The body also adapts, improving its tolerance to heat, optimizing thermoregulation, and increasing sweating efficiency in hot environments. Dry sauna also activates heat shock proteins, responsible for promoting cellular repair and longevity, without the risk of hyperthermia. Unlike a steam sauna, there is no release of vapor containing chemical byproducts such as chlorine, fluoride, and trihalomethanes, making the environment purer, nontoxic, and safer for routine use.

To maximize the benefits of sauna, there are some strategies that can be applied to enhance its effects:

- Proper hydration: sauna causes the body to lose fluids through sweating. To optimize the benefits of sauna and avoid dehydration, it is essential to drink water with unrefined salt before, during, and after the session.

- Regular sessions: studies indicate that cardiovascular and longevity benefits are more associated with regular sauna sessions, ideally 3 to 4 times per week. Continuous practice allows the body to adapt to the heat and improve its biological responses.
- Proper timing: sauna sessions should not be too long. Generally, sessions of 15 to 20 minutes are effective. Longer exposures may overload the body and cause discomfort.
- Alternating between cold and heat: some practices combine sauna sessions with cold baths or immersion in ice water. This alternation between heat and cold may improve circulation and reduce muscle inflammation.

Although sauna is not a curative therapy for cancer, there are studies suggesting that exposure to heat may have protective effects in the fight against cancer, mainly because of the effects of inducing thermal stress in cells. More research is certainly needed, but some preliminary studies indicate that sauna may have an indirect role in cancer prevention, helping reduce associated risk factors, such as exposure to oxidative stress, chronic inflammation, and mitochondrial dysfunction.

In addition, sauna may help relieve symptoms related to cancer treatment, such as muscle pain and fatigue, especially in patients undergoing treatments such as chemotherapy.

Exposure to heat may help to:

- Increase the expression of heat shock proteins, HSPs, which protect cells against stress, including stress caused by radiation or other carcinogenic agents.

- Improve immune function: by stimulating the production of HSPs and other biological mediators, sauna may strengthen the immune system, helping the body fight tumor cells or preventing tumor formation.
- Reduce inflammation: chronic inflammation is one of the factors associated with cancer. Sauna, by reducing inflammation, may help lower the risk of cancer.

As we saw earlier, sauna and heat therapy have many health benefits, ranging from cellular protection and increased longevity to improved cardiovascular health and support for detoxification. Regular practice can stimulate the production of heat shock proteins, which help protect cells from stress and maintain long-term health. Sauna can be a powerful complement for improving quality of life and helping combat various chronic diseases. However, like any therapeutic intervention, it is important to use it properly and integrate it into a healthy lifestyle.

Putting It Into Practice:

- If possible, do one dry sauna session per week.
- If you are already a regular practitioner of this habit, how do you feel afterward? Evaluate whether the duration and hydration are adequate.
- If you do not have access to a sauna, simulate a similar response by increasing body temperature through exercise and observe the effects.

CHAPTER 8

OFF-LABEL THERAPIES AND EMERGING SUBSTANCES

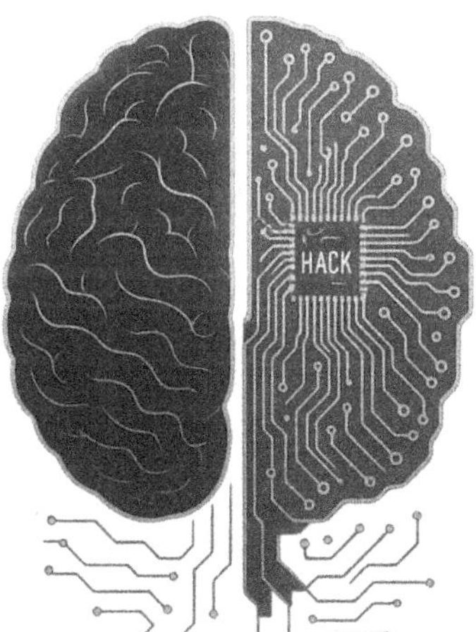

She was diagnosed at a young age with an inflammatory bowel disease that, over the years, doctors classified at times as ulcerative colitis and at other times as Crohn's disease. She went through immunosuppressants, corticosteroids, strict diets, and periods of uncertainty. Through highs and lows, she found in low-dose naltrexone, known as LDN, a turning point: days of intestinal calm, renewed energy, and even moments when remission was considered. There were phases when it seemed she had achieved full balance, with a healthy intestine, no blood, no mucus, and no pain. However, real life did not offer the same absolute control. Wine at social gatherings, bread and pizza shared with family, daily stress, and somewhat restless young children fluctuated as silent triggers that reminded her of the fragility of her condition.

Even so, with each relapse there also came proof of strength. Between CrossFit, strength training, supplements, and dietary adjustments, she learned to recognize the impact of each choice on her body. LDN remained a central ally, allowing periods of stability that had once seemed impossible. The story of this patient, Isabel Fernandes, is the story of someone who, even without achieving perfect control, experienced remarkable progress with low-dose naltrexone, showing that remission can be a tangible horizon when science, discipline, and lifestyle awareness move forward together.

The term "off-label therapies" refers to the use of medications or substances for treatments different from those for which they were originally approved by health authorities, such as the FDA, U.S. Food and Drug Administration, or ANVISA, Brazil's National Health Surveillance Agency. In other words, a substance may be prescribed for a purpose different from the one indicated on its label, based on scientific studies or clinical observations suggesting that it may be effective for another condition. In the context of modern health, some off-label therapies, such as low-dose naltrexone, LDN, methylene blue, GLP-1 and GIP analogs, metformin, minoxidil, ivermectin, T3 or triiodothyronine, high-dose vitamin D, fenbendazole, and acetylsalicylic acid, aspirin, are being explored for their potential benefits beyond those originally anticipated. Next, we will explore these off-label therapies mentioned above.

Low-dose naltrexone, LDN, refers to the use of naltrexone in very low doses, generally between 1 and 4.5 mg, well below the typical dose used to treat opioid dependence, which is 50 mg or more.

Naltrexone is a medication originally approved to treat dependence on opioids and alcohol. It works by blocking opioid receptors in the brain, preventing opioids from binding to those receptors and causing psychoactive effects.

When administered in low doses, LDN appears to have a different effect. Instead of completely blocking opioid receptors, it modulates the immune system and increases the production of endorphins and enkephalins, which are neurotransmitters responsible for pain modulation and immune response.

"Low-dose naltrexone, LDN, may well be the most important therapeutic breakthrough in more than fifty years. It provides a new, safe, and inexpensive method of medical treatment by mobilizing the natural defenses of the immune system itself." David Gluck, MD

LDN has been used off-label to treat a variety of conditions, especially autoimmune diseases and conditions associated with chronic inflammation, such as multiple sclerosis, fibromyalgia, Crohn's disease, among others. Its effect on immune-system modulation may be beneficial in conditions in which the immune system is dysregulated and attacking the body's healthy tissues. In addition, there is some evidence that LDN may reduce chronic inflammation, a common factor in many modern diseases and one of the main causes of many health conditions, such as heart and metabolic diseases.

The drug naltrexone was approved by the FDA in 1984, more than 40 years ago, at a dose of 50 mg with the goal of helping patients with heroin or opium dependence by inhibiting the effect of those drugs. By blocking opioid receptors, naltrexone also blocks the reception of the opioid hormones our brain and adrenal glands produce: beta-endorphin and metenkephalin. Many tissues in the body have receptors for these endorphins and enkephalins, including virtually all the cells of the body's immune system.

In 1981, researchers Patricia McLaughlin and Ian Zagon of Penn State began studies showing how small doses of naltrexone could slow tumor growth in animals. A few years later, in 1985, New York physician Bernard Bihari discovered that a low dose of the substance, about 3 mg administered at night, had an important effect on the human immune system, even improving the response of patients with HIV, the virus that causes AIDS. Later, he established that the ideal dosage for adults would be 4.5 mg. By the mid-1990s, Bihari observed that cancer patients, such as those with lymphoma and pancreatic cancer, could also benefit significantly from the use of LDN. In addition, he found that people with autoimmune diseases, such as lupus, often showed almost immediate control of disease activity when using this therapy.

Although more research is still needed on the long-term effects of LDN, preliminary studies and clinical reports suggest that it has great therapeutic potential, especially for diseases in which inflammation and autoimmunity are involved.

Methylene blue, MB, is already known in the medical field as an antiseptic medication and is used to treat methemoglobinemia, a rare blood disorder that reduces the blood's ability to carry oxygen and may be hereditary or acquired. Manufactured in 1876, it was used to treat malaria after it was found to have antimicrobial properties. It is also used as a dye to stain certain parts of the body before or during surgery.

It is a substance that traditionally was used as a dye and as a medication to treat cyanide poisoning and other conditions. In recent years, it has been studied for its potential to optimize mitochondrial function and promote neuroprotection, making it a powerful nootropic in the biohacking world.

Few people know this, but my experience with methylene blue began unexpectedly within the world of competitive CrossFit. This sport demands the maximum from the human body: three or four days of intense events in which the athlete goes to the physical and mental limit. But what came afterward was a problem: many of these elite athletes spent the following week in bed, worn down, often with throat infections and a brutal drop in immunity. It was as though the body collected the price of performance. It was in that setting that methylene blue entered the game. As a reducing agent, it improves mitochondrial efficiency and enhances ATP production, the energy currency of our cells. But in clinical practice we discovered it went far beyond that. As a powerful antioxidant, immunomodulator, and even antiviral, it completely changed the outcome for these athletes. With the introduction of this off-label therapy, we stopped seeing our champions succumb to infections after competitions. Instead of spending days in bed, they were back to training in record time, maintaining performance without paying the price of immune collapse. It was like flipping a switch: dominating not only inside the arena, but also in recovery.

Methylene blue, which had once seemed like merely a curious laboratory dye, became a strategic ally in high-performance medicine. And today, in the office, it is not just another substance, but the difference between winning the championship and winning the post-championship as well.

Proper mitochondrial function is crucial for cellular health and the prevention of cellular aging.

The substance may also improve the oxidative capacity of cells, helping improve the use of oxygen by cells and reduce the production of free radicals, which may decrease oxidative stress and thereby protect nerve cells, neuroprotection.

In terms of neuroprotection, methylene blue has been studied as a potential therapy for neurodegenerative diseases, such as Alzheimer's disease and Parkinson's disease, in which it could play a role through inhibitory effects on Tau protein aggregation and on the formation and deposition of beta-amyloid peptide, in addition to its ability to reduce oxidative damage in brain cells and promote brain mitochondrial health.

It may help protect brain cells against damage caused by oxidative stress, which is particularly relevant in neurodegenerative diseases. There is also mitochondrial support, because by improving mitochondrial function, methylene blue may be useful in the treatment of age-related conditions, as well as in optimizing cellular energy production in various types of cells.

More study is still needed regarding the long-term benefits and the precise mechanisms of action, but methylene blue has attracted considerable interest as a potential neuroprotective therapy and an aid in cellular longevity.

We also have acetylsalicylic acid, better known as aspirin or baby aspirin, which is a medication widely used to relieve pain, reduce fever, and reduce inflammation. In recent years, it has also been investigated for its potential role in longevity and cardiovascular risk reduction, especially in low doses.

In 2013, Bloomberg reported an analysis by Risk Management Solutions showing how a simple tablet could generate a multi-billion-dollar impact on the economy: the daily use of aspirin, by reducing cancer risk and increasing survival, could raise pension costs in the United States and Europe by as much as 100 billion dollars. The logic was clear: by prolonging the lives of millions of people, a cheap and accessible drug would end up putting pressure on pension systems, creating a paradox in which a public-health medical advance would become a global economic challenge. The justification is that studies published in The Lancet showed that daily doses of aspirin reduce the risk of developing or dying from cancer and inhibit tumor spread.

How does it work? Aspirin works by inhibiting the cyclooxygenase enzyme, COX, which is responsible for the production of prostaglandins, substances that play a crucial role in inflammation and in the formation of blood clots.

In low doses, aspirin has been widely used to prevent strokes and myocardial infarctions. It helps reduce clot formation, lowering the risk of arterial blockages that can lead to these conditions, and it has also been studied as a possible intervention to prevent certain types of cancer, such as colon cancer.

Aspirin may help reduce chronic inflammation, one of the main risk factors for chronic diseases associated with aging, such as heart disease, type 2 diabetes, and cancer.

Aspirin, once metabolized into salicylic acid, exerts a potent anti-inflammatory effect that directly contributes to improving insulin resistance. This metabolite inhibits the inflammatory NF-κB pathway and reduces the activity of the IKKβ enzyme, responsible for blocking insulin signaling in cells. As a result, there is a reduction in chronic low-grade inflammation, a central factor in the pathophysiology of insulin resistance, promoting greater glucose uptake and improved cellular insulin sensitivity. Interestingly, in old newspapers it is possible to find records of aspirin being used in the treatment of glycosuria, something that today we understand as a reflection of its action on the inflammatory mechanisms that interfere with glucose metabolism. These effects, now better understood, make aspirin a promising molecule in the treatment of metabolic syndrome and type 2 diabetes. So why does aspirin continue to be prescribed mostly to people who are obese, elderly, sedentary, or have heart disease? As a biohacker therapy, we indicate aspirin from youth onward, in low doses of 81 mg daily or every other day. There is no need to wait until you get sick to consider aspirin an option; ideally, we should anticipate and place it as something preventive and of immeasurable value for longevity by preventing chronic diseases such as diabetes and cancer itself.

It is important to emphasize that regular aspirin use should be done under medical supervision. Always seek guidance, and I want to make it very clear that what I am discussing here is for your information and knowledge, not as a basis for self-medication.

These off-label therapies and emerging substances have significant potential to improve health and increase longevity, but their use must be carefully monitored, especially at nontraditional doses or for conditions not officially approved.

Low-dose naltrexone, LDN, methylene blue, and acetylsalicylic acid are just a few examples of how substances approved for specific uses are being explored to treat a broad range of conditions, from chronic inflammation to neurodegenerative diseases and heart problems.

The history of off-label therapies is a testimony to how the history of medicine is written by methods and paths that, even when manipulated and directed by the financial side, cannot hide the fact that great possibilities, outcomes, and accidental findings, even when discovered and often ignored, do not go unnoticed by physicians with a humanitarian, functional, and integrative outlook.

That is how aspirin, created as a simple analgesic in the nineteenth century, ended up revealing itself as the greatest ally against heart attacks and strokes; how sildenafil, frustrated as a vasodilator for angina, became Viagra, a symbol of sexual potency and later a vital treatment against pulmonary hypertension; or how minoxidil, from a discontinued oral antihypertensive, became a source of hope against baldness by unexpectedly restoring hair in patients with androgenetic alopecia. The same happened with bupropion, an antidepressant that showed it could free smokers from their dependence, and with metformin, which crossed generations to be studied today as a candidate longevity drug, increasing AMPK and bringing more cellular energy.

Methylene blue, once merely a laboratory dye and even a weapon against malaria, now reappears as a mitochondrial modulator and possible neuronal protector against degenerative diseases. Ivermectin, discovered in Japanese soil and awarded the Nobel Prize for freeing entire communities from river blindness, opened the way for investigations as an immunomodulator and antiviral, reportedly exceptional in defense against COVID-19.

Rapamycin, born from the remote soil of Easter Island, traveled from antibiotic to immunosuppressant in transplants and today is seen as one of the most promising molecules against aging. Lithium carbonate, which in small concentrations in water was already associated with lower suicide risk, returned in minimal doses as a mood stabilizer and possible neuroprotector against the aluminum present in vaccines and water. Ketamine, used as an anesthetic in battlefields, has reemerged as one of the fastest therapies against treatment-resistant depression. Even fenbendazole, known only as a veterinary antihelminthic, found a place in discussions of experimental oncology, showing that the boundary between the unlikely and the revolutionary is thin.

These examples show that clinical boldness, when guided by prudence and an attentive eye, is capable of transforming side effects into opportunities and therapeutic failures into brilliant discoveries. Ultimately, off-label uses reveal that each drug is more than the label it carries, it is an invitation to think beyond, a reminder that medicine does not end with protocols, but renews itself in the meeting between science, art, and courage.

I advise you to research off-label therapy further and reflect on whether any of them make sense for you. If you are interested in any of them, talk to your doctor or a healthcare professional to better understand their risks and benefits.

CHAPTER 9

GROUNDING AND ELECTROMAGNETISM

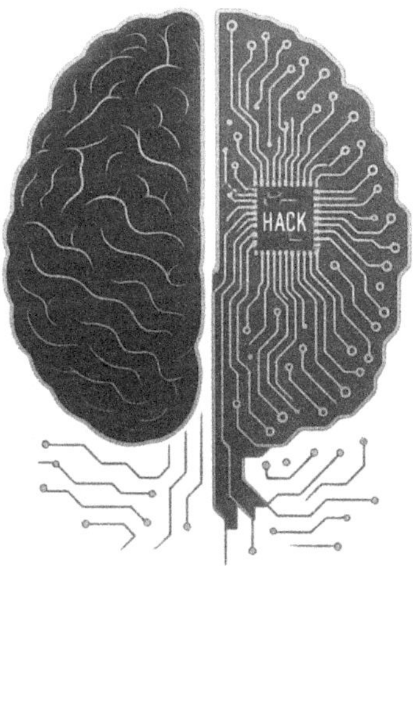

There was a time when human beings lived in direct contact with the earth, walking barefoot, sleeping on the ground, cultivating and harvesting with their own hands. That contact was natural, part of life itself. But when rubber soles appeared in footwear, that bond was broken. Rubber insulates, and we stopped receiving what the earth had always given us: vital electricity. The human body functions as an electrical system. When we are not connected to the ground, we accumulate excessive positive charge, we become filled with protons. It is as if the body were too charged, with no way to discharge. Grounding restores balance, because the earth is full of free electrons, ready to neutralize that excess and bring cellular harmony.

These electrons do not appear by chance. The earth is constantly recharged by lightning that comes down from the sky during storms, loading the soil with energy. That energy is as essential as the nutrients, vitamins, and minerals that nourish us. In the same way that we need food to nourish the physical body, we need the earth's electrons to nourish the electrical body. Because, deep down, we are energy too.

Grounding, also called earthing, is the practice of reconnecting the human body directly to the earth's energy, whether by walking barefoot on grass, sand, or soil, or by using tools that conduct this natural force, such as grounding mats, sheets, pillowcases, bracelets, and mattresses with conductive wires connected to the ground wire. More than a simple habit, it is a reunion with the vitality, balance, and spirituality that spring from genuine contact with the soil.

When we talk about grounding, many people think only of walking barefoot on grass or sand. But the concept is broader and grounded in science. The earth's soil has a constant negative electrical charge, made up of billions of free electrons, continually renewed by atmospheric discharges. When the human body comes into contact with that conductive surface, those electrons are transferred into the body, neutralizing the excess protons and reactive oxygen species that we accumulate daily because of stress, pollution, and electromagnetic exposure. This simple exchange of charges has documented effects in studies: reduced inflammation, improved sleep, balanced cortisol, and restored heart rate variability. But it is not only direct contact through the feet with the ground that promotes this balance. A waterfall bath, for example, works like immersion in a conductive field, allowing the immediate passage of electrons to the skin. Sunlight, in turn, not only triggers vitamin D production, but also carries photons that interact with our mitochondria, optimizing ATP production and strengthening the endogenous antioxidant system.

Practices such as meditation and deep breathing also act as forms of grounding. Studies in neuroscience show that breath control modulates the vagus nerve and the autonomic nervous system, reducing sympathetic tone and inducing greater cardiac coherence. From a bioelectrical standpoint, that is just as fundamental as receiving electrons from the soil, because it reorganizes internal electrical charge and restores balance to the body.

Grounding, therefore, is not an esoteric or folkloric concept. It is pure physiology: the Earth, permanently charged by lightning and storms, offers an inexhaustible source of vital electrical energy. We, as bioelectrical organisms, need that flow just as we need vitamins, minerals, and nutrients. Ignoring this was one of modernity's greatest deviations, when we began isolating our bodies with rubber soles, raised houses, and routines disconnected from nature. Recovering this practice is recovering health in its deepest dimension: cellular, energetic, and spiritual.

Electromagnetic fields, EMFs, are present in our daily lives through electronic devices, Wi-Fi networks, power transmission lines, and telecommunications towers. Studies indicate that prolonged exposure may have biological effects, including sleep changes, increased oxidative stress, and impacts on cellular function.

Exposure to artificial electromagnetic fields generated by electronic devices, cell towers, and electrical grids, all abundant in our day, may be associated with symptoms such as fatigue, headaches, sleep disturbances, and changes in the immune system. Proper grounding may contribute to reducing these effects by dissipating unwanted electrical charges from the body.

When we do not ground ourselves, especially when wearing shoes with rubber soles, we isolate ourselves from the earth's natural electrical charge. This isolation may intensify the negative effects of EMFs on the body. Grounding, by allowing the transfer of electrons between our body and the ground, helps neutralize free radicals and may reduce inflammation.

Several studies indicate that chronic exposure to low-intensity electromagnetic fields, such as Wi-Fi, cell towers, and electronic devices that emit non-ionizing radiation, may induce a significant increase in reactive oxygen species, ROS, within cells, with peroxynitrite, ONOO, being one of the main mediators of damage. The mechanism described involves activation of voltage-gated calcium channels, VGCCs, which promotes greater intracellular Ca^{2+} entry. This excess calcium stimulates enzymes such as nitric oxide synthase, NOS, increasing nitric oxide, NO, production, which, when reacting with superoxide, O_2^-, forms peroxynitrite.

This highly oxidizing molecule is capable of damaging lipids, proteins, DNA, and mitochondria, triggering inflammation and cellular dysfunction associated with fatigue, chronic pain, sleep disorders, neuroinflammation, and diseases related to environmental exposure. This line of reasoning was widely explored by researcher Martin Pall, PhD, in his reviews, in which he demonstrates how activation of VGCCs and the resulting increase in peroxynitrite constitute a central pathway of oxidative and inflammatory stress caused by electromagnetic pollution.

Studies show that spending time in nature and practicing grounding bring various health benefits. Direct contact with the earth, sand, grass, soil, may improve sleep quality, reduce pain, and strengthen the immune system. Although there is no exact defined amount of time to maximize these benefits, research suggests that at least 20 minutes of grounding per day may generate positive effects.

In 2010, a study from UFMG analyzed cancer mortality in Belo Horizonte, capital of Minas Gerais, the city where I live in Brazil, and found that more than 80% of deaths occurred in people living within 500 meters of cell towers. The work, done using geoprocessing, showed that the shorter the distance from the tower, the higher the mortality rate, suggesting a concerning relationship between electromagnetic pollution and cancer risk.

For those who live in urban environments, where direct contact with the earth is limited, there are alternatives such as grounding mats and mattresses. These devices are connected to an electrical grounding point and simulate the effect of being barefoot on the earth.

EMF blockers include fabrics, paints, and stickers designed to reduce exposure to electromagnetic fields. Although there is still debate over the effectiveness of these products, many people report improvements in sleep quality and reduced fatigue symptoms after using them.

Some strategies for reducing the impact of EMFs include walking barefoot on the ground whenever possible, avoiding sleeping near Wi-Fi routers and electronic devices, which is why it is important to keep your bedroom free of electronics at night. Try to reduce screen time and take regular breaks to minimize exposure to magnetic fields.

Other tools that may minimize the effects of electromagnetic pollution include:

- Red light and near-infrared therapy, PBM: increases cytochrome c oxidase activity, improves mitochondrial function and ATP production, reducing cellular vulnerability to oxidative stress.
- Deep and restorative sleep: essential for melatonin, one of the most powerful endogenous antioxidants, which also acts as a protector against EMF-related damage.
- Vitamin C: a water-soluble antioxidant that neutralizes free radicals in plasma and protects cellular membranes.
- Curcumin: a natural inflammatory modulator that reduces NF-κB and protects against oxidative damage.
- Magnesium: regulates calcium entry into VGCC channels, functioning as a natural blocker of this central EMF-damage pathway.
- Selenium and zinc: cofactors of antioxidant enzymes such as glutathione peroxidase and superoxide dismutase, strengthening endogenous defenses.
- Omega-3: stabilizes cellular membranes and reduces systemic inflammation.
- Adaptogens, ashwagandha, rhodiola, ginseng: help modulate the HPA axis, reducing vulnerability to environmental stress.

Biohacking Tools Against Electromagnetic Pollution

- Grounding: direct transfer of free electrons from the earth to neutralize positive charges.
- Environmental shielding: the use of fabrics, paints, curtains, and clothing with conductive fibers that attenuate exposure to electromagnetic waves.
- Digital hygiene: turning off Wi-Fi at night, keeping your phone away from your body, and preferring calls with wired headphones.
- Exposure to nature: ocean, waterfalls, forests, and sunlight, which provide electrons, photons, and negative ions.
- Cold baths and sauna: increase the expression of heat shock proteins, HSPs, improving cellular resilience.
- Deep breathing and meditation: modulate the vagus nerve and reduce systemic oxidative stress, complementing the body's defenses.

One of the tools I have adopted in my routine is molecular hydrogen inhalation. I try to do this protocol three times a week, in sessions lasting about an hour. Inhaled H_2 works as a selective antioxidant, neutralizing highly aggressive radicals such as the hydroxyl radical and peroxynitrite, which are directly linked to oxidative stress generated by electromagnetic pollution. By reducing the formation of reactive species and modulating inflammatory pathways such as NF-κB, TNF-α, and IL-6, it protects my mitochondria, cellular membranes, and DNA. I often say it does not block radiation, but it greatly reduces the biological impact it causes.

In addition, I use a grounding mat from the Hooga brand, which I bought on Amazon, and in my living room I keep orgonites, crystals, and a large amethyst stone. All of this is meant to support my electrical balance. I also try to stimulate my autonomic nervous system with Pulsetto and vagus nerve activation exercises. Sunlight is part of my treatment: I run outdoors, shirtless, at least three times a week to receive electrons and solar energy directly on my skin. At night, I always turn off the Wi-Fi to reduce the electromagnetic load inside the house. And, as a foundation, I constantly work on my minerals, using supplements and also unrefined salt with water to keep the body electrically well nourished.

The combination of grounding and protective measures against electromagnetic fields may be an effective strategy for improving health and overall well-being in an increasingly digitalized world.

Putting It Into Practice:

- Spend 20 minutes a day barefoot on soil, grass, or damp sand.
- Reduce your exposure to electromagnetic fields by turning off the Wi-Fi at night or keeping your phone away from your body while you sleep.

CHAPTER 10

THE IMPORTANCE OF SUNLIGHT AND CIRCADIAN REGULATION

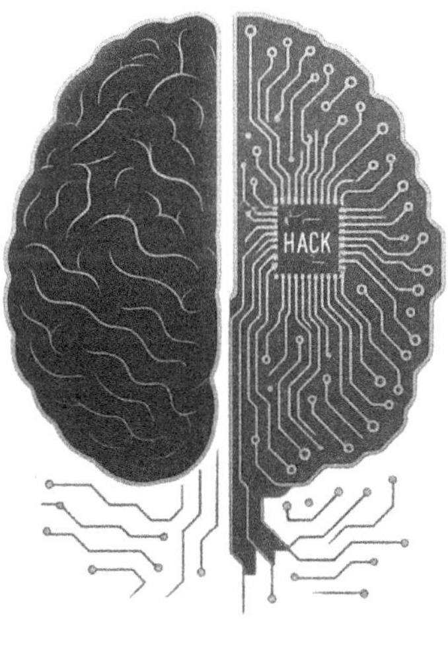

The use of light in the treatment of disease has been reported since Ancient Greece. Initially called "heliotherapy," it involved exposing the sick to sunlight to heal their illnesses.

For millennia, sunlight was seen as a powerful ally of health. Long before modern medicine, ancient peoples already recognized the restorative effects of sun exposure. In the late nineteenth and early twentieth centuries, this practice was refined in clinics called solariums, where patients with tuberculosis, rickets, and other illnesses were treated with heliotherapy, that is, therapeutic exposure to sunlight. During the 1918 Spanish flu pandemic, the use of light as therapy, called "phototherapy," was identified as one of the most significant factors in reducing mortality.

There are striking photographic records of these institutions, with rows of beds outdoors or on sun-drenched porches, where the sick recovered not only through the direct action of light, but also through natural alignment with the rhythms of day and night.

However, with the advance of urbanization and life in enclosed environments, a true heliophobia emerged, the fear of the sun. Encouraged by exaggerated campaigns about the risks of skin cancer, this aversion was intensified by the indiscriminate use of sunscreens. Despite the importance of these products in specific contexts, many contain chemical substances such as oxybenzone and octinoxate, which not only interfere with vitamin D production, but also have potential hormone-disrupting effects.

Most sunscreens do not protect against UVA rays, the skin-aging rays that are associated with cancers such as melanoma.

Sunscreen should be understood as a medical tool, not as a shield for living hidden from the sun. We spend most of our time hidden from sunlight, exposed to artificial lights and protected by glass, acrylic, and films that block much of the radiation.

Sunscreen mainly protects against UVB rays, which are responsible for producing vitamin D, and many formulas fail to provide adequate protection against UVA rays, which make up most of the radiation that reaches us, penetrate deeply into the skin, cause premature aging, and are closely linked to melanoma. That is why it is not enough to look only at the SPF. It measures defense against UVB and should be at least 30, while UVA protection is evaluated by the PPD, which needs to be at least 20, something still neglected by most brands.

Another critical point is that many traditional chemical sunscreens use substances such as oxybenzone, octinoxate, homosalate, and octocrylene, which act as endocrine disruptors, mimicking hormones such as estrogen and interfering with metabolic and reproductive processes and even with the risk of hormone-dependent cancer. For that reason, the most responsible guidance is not the indiscriminate use of sunscreen, but rather balance: moderate and intelligent sun exposure to ensure vitamin D synthesis and circadian regulation, and the use of quality sunscreens, preferably physical ones, based on zinc oxide and non-nano titanium dioxide, which offer a safe barrier against UVA and UVB without compromising the endocrine system.

Sun exposure goes far beyond vitamin D synthesis. Sunlight, especially the blue light present in the early hours of the day, acts as a powerful synchronizer of our biological clock, the so-called circadian rhythm. Circadian rhythm is the name given to the internal "biological clock" that regulates almost all the functions of our body in a cycle of approximately 24 hours. It is controlled mainly by exposure to light and darkness, but it is also influenced by meal timing, physical activity, and even temperature.

This internal clock regulates fundamental processes such as sleep, hormone secretion, such as cortisol and melatonin, body temperature, and energy metabolism. Dysregulation of this system has been associated with disorders such as depression, obesity, type 2 diabetes, and cardiovascular disease. Satchidananda, Satchin, Panda, a researcher at the Salk Institute and a global authority in chronobiology, is known for showing how circadian cycles regulate virtually all biological functions, from gene expression to energy metabolism.

In fact, studies show that people who get sun exposure in the morning have more stable cortisol levels, better sleep quality, and a lower risk of developing depression. Natural light also positively affects mitochondrial function. This happens because certain wavelengths of light, such as near infrared, stimulate the activity of cytochrome c oxidase, a key enzyme in ATP production, our main cellular energy currency.

In a world where we spend more than 90% of our time indoors, it is essential to restore conscious contact with natural light. The greatest mistake of the modern lifestyle is the disruption of this synchrony: we work in closed environments without natural light, we use screens at night that confuse the biological clock, and we eat outside the ideal metabolic window, which dysregulates hormones, sleep, energy, and increases the risk of chronic diseases.

Some practical strategies for realigning yourself with the solar cycle can help, such as morning sun exposure. Seek natural light as soon as you wake up and stay there for 10 to 30 minutes. This helps regulate circadian rhythm, stabilizes mood, and prepares our body for the day. Whenever possible, eat lunch outside or take sun breaks. Even on cloudy days, natural light is much more intense and beneficial than indoor lighting. Reduce the use of screens and intense white lights after sunset. Use amber or red lights, which have less impact on melatonin production. Prefer physical sunscreens, with zinc oxide or titanium dioxide, avoid excessive exposure during peak sun hours, but do not completely prevent contact with light. These are simple strategies anyone can follow, and they will certainly contribute greatly to your health.

With the introduction of electric light, we artificially extended the day, and that brought consequences. Chronic exposure to blue light at night suppresses melatonin production, harming sleep and affecting the immune system. In addition, continuous artificial lighting can desynchronize internal rhythms, creating a state of "social jet lag" even without changing time zones. Simple interventions, such as using blue-light filters on screens or installing warm lights at night, can mitigate this impact.

Let us understand a little more about how circadian regulation happens. Imagine that inside every cell in your body, there is a small biological clock. This clock does not work in isolation. It is synchronized to a "central pacemaker," located in the suprachiasmatic nucleus, SCN, of the hypothalamus, which receives direct information from the retina through specialized ganglion cells capable of detecting mainly morning blue light. From this signal, the SCN adjusts the other clocks in the body, ensuring that the entire organism functions in harmony with the cycle of light and darkness over approximately 24 hours, hence the name circadian, from the Latin circa diem, meaning "about a day."

Circadian regulation coordinates hundreds of physiological processes, among them: the release of hormones such as cortisol, melatonin, insulin, and growth hormone, regulation of body temperature, contribution to sleep phases, wakefulness, light sleep, deep sleep, REM, assistance in regulating hunger and appetite, and cellular repair and gene expression. At the molecular level, the SCN regulates the so-called clock genes, such as CLOCK, BMAL1, PER, Period, and CRY, Cryptochrome. These genes interact in feedback loops: CLOCK and BMAL1 activate the expression of PER and CRY, which then inhibit their own activation, creating oscillations of about 24 hours. This mechanism generates rhythmic pulses that control the transcription of thousands of genes throughout the body.

When this clock is aligned with the natural cycle of light and darkness, that is, when we wake up at sunrise, eat at consistent times, and sleep shortly after nightfall, the body operates in harmony. But in the modern world, we are constantly sending conflicting signals to our circadian system: artificial light at night, mistimed eating, irregular sleep, jet lag, screen use, and lack of morning sunlight exposure.

This mismatch is called circadian dysrhythmia, and it is strongly associated with metabolic and inflammatory disorders and even cancer. The World Health Organization, WHO, has even classified night shift work as "potentially carcinogenic" because of chronic circadian dysregulation. Night shift work is one of the greatest factors of circadian dysregulation in the modern world. The International Agency for Research on Cancer, IARC/WHO, classified night shift work as "probably carcinogenic to humans," Group 2A, due to strong evidence that chronic melatonin suppression and circadian dysregulation favor mutations and cellular proliferation. Examples of shift-work professions include healthcare workers, such as on-call physicians and nurses, bus drivers, police officers, pilots and air traffic controllers, security guards, and any 24-hour support job.

Light is the main synchronizing agent of our internal clock, a phenomenon called zeitgeber, a German term meaning "time giver." But not just any light: the intensity, spectrum, and timing of exposure make all the difference.

Morning blue light is the most efficient light for suppressing melatonin and stimulating wakefulness. It activates our biological clock, regulates morning cortisol, and sets the circadian rhythm for the new day. Darkness is equally important. When the retina no longer perceives blue light, the pineal gland begins to release melatonin, the sleep hormone, which also acts as an antioxidant, anti-inflammatory, and immune regulator.

That is why being exposed to bright artificial light after sunset, such as LED lamps and electronic screens, misleads the brain, delaying melatonin production and thereby affecting the entire nighttime recovery cycle.

Chronodisruption is the chronic dysregulation of circadian rhythms, which are the physical and mental changes that occur over about 24 hours. This dysregulation can create a true domino effect in the body. For example, if the cortisol peak occurs too late, due to nighttime light exposure, it can compete with melatonin, making sleep more difficult and increasing stress. Insulin sensitivity is naturally higher in the morning and lower at night. Eating late at night, therefore, increases the chance of glucose spikes and fat accumulation. Sleep deprivation dysregulates these two hormones related to satiety and appetite, contributing to binge eating and weight gain. Testosterone and GH, growth hormone, are both released mainly during deep sleep. When sleep is shortened or fragmented, the production of these hormones is severely compromised, affecting muscle recovery, metabolism, and even mood.

When we talk about sunlight, it is common to think about tanned skin, vitamin D, and the sense of well-being we feel when walking under the open sky. But there is an even deeper phenomenon happening at the cellular level: the interaction between light and mitochondria, the true power plants of our body.

Sunlight literally feeds the mitochondria, improving the cells' energy performance. Michael Hamblin, a Harvard researcher and global authority in photobiomodulation, argues that controlled exposure to red and infrared light can help with neurodegenerative diseases, chronic pain, inflammation, and even depression.

Hormone production is also deeply connected to the solar cycle and to the energetic state of cells. Testosterone and luteinizing hormone, LH, essential for reproductive health and vitality, show greater production when there is more sun exposure, something already observed in studies on seasonal variation. Melatonin, besides regulating sleep, has antioxidant action in the mitochondria. It is synthesized from serotonin, which in turn depends on exposure to natural light. Without morning light, serotonin falls. Without serotonin, there is no melatonin at night. Cortisol, our "wake-up" hormone, should reach its peak right at sunrise. This peak is not only a response to waking up, it is stimulated by the light entering through the retina.

With well-functioning mitochondria, the body has enough energy to maintain hormonal balance, regenerate tissues, fight inflammation, and sustain cognitive functions. When they function poorly, the body enters "energy-saving mode," increasing fatigue, weight gain, anxiety, and degenerative processes.

The influence of sunlight also reaches the brain. Morning exposure to natural light increases the release of dopamine and serotonin, neurotransmitters associated with mood, motivation, and a sense of well-being. That is why it is no coincidence that depression rates rise in regions with long winters and little light, a condition known as Seasonal Affective Disorder, SAD.

Studies show that just 30 minutes of natural light in the morning can significantly increase serotonin production. White-light therapy, 10,000 lux, for example, is used clinically to treat SAD, but it is only a simulation of what the sun naturally does.

Nature never separated human health from sunlight. It is only in recent history that we began to fear it, hiding ourselves inside closed homes, cars with dark windows, and artificially lit offices. The result? An epidemic of fatigue, insomnia, hormonal imbalances, and silent chronic diseases.

Restoring contact with the sun, consciously, safely, and daily, is not merely a healthy habit. It is a way of reactivating our ancestral biology, reconnecting with natural time, and recovering an energy that literally comes from the sky.

Knowledge without action is like the sun that does not rise: it is there, but it does not illuminate. After everything we have explored about the importance of sunlight, circadian rhythms, and cellular energy, it is time to turn theory into practice. And the good news is that there is no need to change your whole life, only your rhythm.

Even those who live in large cities, with little time outdoors, can apply simple and effective strategies to reconnect with the natural cycles of light.

When I talk about circadian rhythm with my patients, I explain that sleeping well is not something solved only at night, at bedtime. The cycle is built throughout the day, and your lifestyle influences it 100%. In my daily life, I apply this practically: first thing in the morning, I expose myself to natural sunlight for at least 20 minutes. This simple act of opening the bedroom windows is like flipping the switch on the circadian cycle, initiating the natural synchronization process of all the body's biological clocks. In addition, I like to take a cold shower, which awakens my dopaminergic axis, releases adrenaline, norepinephrine, and cortisol physiologically, and prepares my mind and body for wakefulness. This morning routine creates the foundation so that, at night, the body knows it is time to shut down.

At night, sleep hygiene becomes a sacred ritual. The bedroom needs to be completely dark, because even minimal light is enough to inhibit melatonin production, the essential hormone for initiating and maintaining deep sleep. If there are outside noises, I use earplugs or white noise. The bed is meant only for sleep or intimacy, never for cell phone use, television, or work. Three hours before bedtime, I begin reducing mental stimuli, slowing the mind down, avoiding solving problems or planning the next day. I also avoid nighttime exercise, caffeine after midday, and I use amber-filter glasses designed to block blue light or night mode on electronics when necessary. My goal is to sleep before midnight, preferably by 9:00 p.m., aligned with the physiological melatonin peak, because that is when the body enters a state of deep repair.

Another fundamental point I apply in my life is metabolic preparation: light meals at night, at least two hours before going to bed, prioritizing foods that are easy to digest. During the day, I hydrate my body, but I reduce fluid intake one hour before bed so I do not interrupt my rest with trips to the bathroom. And finally, I always end the day with a calming ritual such as light reading, prayer, worship, or relaxing music to teach my brain to switch off.

I speak often about the importance of achieving at least two hours of deep sleep per night, because it is during this phase that the body releases growth hormone, repairs tissues, consolidates memories, regulates the immune system, and clears toxins accumulated in the brain. When a person experiences this consistently, daily energy multiplies, the mind becomes clearer, insulin resistance improves, hormonal regulation comes into balance, and even mood changes. In other words, deep sleep is one of the simplest and most powerful interventions that exists for changing anyone's health and life.

Circadian rhythm is not a passive event: it is active, physiological, strategic, and must be protected. By applying these strategies consistently, you teach your body to regulate itself in a way no pill can provide.

Exposure to natural light in the early morning hours is perhaps the most powerful action for regulating the biological clock. This simple habit sends a clear signal to your brain: "The day has begun." That adjusts your cortisol peak, improves focus, stabilizes mood, and prepares your body to sleep at the right time at night. Open the windows and go out to the balcony or yard when you wake up. Walk for 10 to 20 minutes outdoors, even if it is cloudy, natural light is still much more intense than artificial light. Avoid dark sunglasses first thing in the morning, because they block the stimulus the retina needs.

Direct sunlight on the body is essential for vitamin D production, nitric oxide synthesis, a natural vasodilator, and mitochondrial stimulation. Small daily doses are more effective, and safer, than long occasional exposures. Have lunch outdoors whenever you can. Expose your arms and legs for at least 15 minutes at midday, or according to what your skin tone allows. Avoid sunscreen during that brief period, but protect yourself when necessary and outside the therapeutic window.

What you do in the two hours before bedtime defines the quality of your sleep. At nightfall, the ideal is to start slowing down, reducing stimuli, and recreating an atmosphere of darkness, as our ancestors had with fire. Lower the intensity of light after 6:00 p.m. Use amber or red bulbs at night. Activate night mode on screens or use apps such as f.lux and Night Shift. If possible, use blue-light-blocking glasses.

The body loves predictability. Eating and sleeping at irregular times creates metabolic disorder, even with a healthy diet. Have breakfast between 6:00 a.m. and 9:00 a.m., with light exposure. Eat your last meal by 8:00 p.m. at the latest. Ideally, try to sleep between 9:30 p.m. and 10:30 p.m., in a dark and quiet environment.

The red light emitted by fire has calming effects and respects nighttime biology. It is no coincidence that human beings have always slept better after hours by the fire. Today we have some modern alternatives, such as lamps with soft red light in the bedroom, candles used safely to slow down at night, and smart lights that change color throughout the day.

Health is not only a matter of what we eat or how much we exercise, but also when we do these things and under what kind of light we live. Light is an invisible nutrient. It regulates hormones, energy, mood, immunity, and sleep. Neglecting it is like trying to grow a plant without sun.

By reclaiming our relationship with the sun, without fear but with awareness, we also reclaim a forgotten part of our nature. In a world that pushes us toward the artificial, reconnecting with the natural is, paradoxically, the greatest act of modernity.

Putting It Into Practice:

- Get 15 minutes of sun in the morning and avoid blue light for at least 1 hour before bed.
- Try using blue-light-blocking glasses or adjust your home lighting in the evening.

CHAPTER 11

SLEEP AND SLEEP HYGIENE

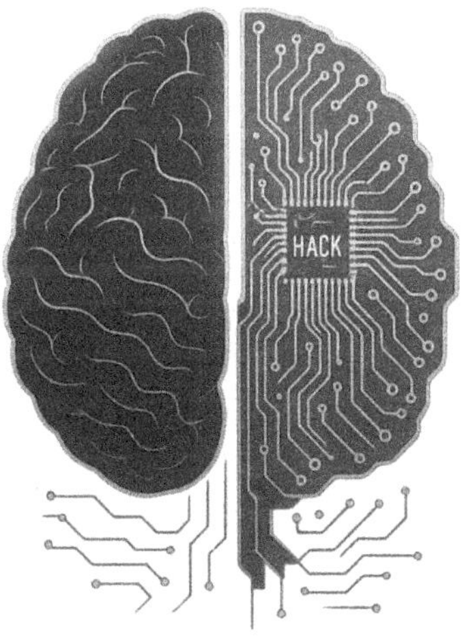

We live in an era that values relentless productivity, the hustle, doing more with less. And among the first things we sacrifice to fit more into the day is sleep. I myself sacrificed many nights of sleep during medical school.

Sleep is often seen as a waste of time, a luxury, or even a weakness. But the truth is that those who do not sleep well do not live well and do not think well. Science today is clear: sleep is not a passive moment of rest, but an active state of repair, consolidation, and renewal. Ignoring it is like paying compound interest with your own physical, emotional, and cognitive health.

Sleep deprivation, whether partial, sleeping less than necessary, or chronic, the accumulation of poorly slept nights, affects practically every system in the human body. Studies show that sleeping less than 6 hours per night is associated with: a higher risk of cardiovascular disease, reduced insulin sensitivity and greater susceptibility to type 2 diabetes, impairment of the immune system with more infections, cognitive deterioration including memory loss, difficulty focusing, and irritability, reduced testosterone and growth hormone production, and a greater risk of Alzheimer's, due to less effective brain cleansing by the glymphatic system.

In addition, sleep deprivation has a cumulative neurobehavioral effect. Matthew Walker, neuroscientist and author of *Why We Sleep*, warns: "You cannot adapt to sleeping less than you need. You only get worse slowly, and stop noticing how bad you feel."

Contrary to popular belief, sleeping well is not just resting. Sleep is the moment when the brain organizes memories and consolidates learning, the body secretes anabolic hormones such as GH and testosterone, the liver enters detox mode, the immune system activates defense cells, and brain synapses adjust themselves, optimizing cognitive functions.

Studies show that people who maintain good sleep quality for decades have a lower risk of chronic disease, better cognitive capacity at age 70 and 80, and greater emotional resilience.

Sleep does not happen by chance. It is orchestrated by a hormonal interplay synchronized with the light-dark cycle of the environment. Two central hormones in this dance are melatonin and cortisol.

Melatonin is considered the hormone of darkness. Produced by the pineal gland in response to the absence of light, melatonin initiates the sleep process and acts as an antioxidant and immune modulator. It signals to the body that it is time to slow down, lowers body temperature, and induces the deeper stages of sleep. Its production is highly sensitive to blue light, which makes screens and LED bulbs at night an invisible saboteur.

Cortisol, on the other hand, is the waking hormone. An antagonist of melatonin, cortisol ideally peaks between 6:00 a.m. and 9:00 a.m., waking the body, regulating metabolism, and preparing the mind for focus and action. When morning light enters the eyes, it suppresses melatonin and stimulates cortisol, restarting the circadian cycle.

When these hormones are out of sync, whether due to insomnia, artificial light at night, or chronic stress, the circadian cycle becomes dysregulated, and deep sleep disappears.

The main tool for optimizing sleep begins with routine, a set of simple and effective practices that significantly improve the quality and depth of your rest. They are small adjustments in your routine that directly affect hormonal regulation, brain function, physical and mental recovery, and also reduce anxiety, depressive symptoms, and increase creativity.

The first thing we need to correct in the patient is sleep. Improving mood and energy depends on a good night of restorative sleep. These practices I am sharing with you here were built on many studies and personal experiences. Take note and, more importantly, put them into practice.

1. Wake up with natural light

As soon as you wake up, open the curtains and windows. Expose yourself to sunlight for at least 20 minutes, even on cloudy days. This helps regulate your biological clock, lowers melatonin levels, and stimulates the release of cortisol and other morning hormones. This simple habit improves mood, increases energy, and starts your day with vitality.

2. Cold shower in the morning

Start the day with a warm shower and finish with cold water. This activates heat shock proteins, improves neurotransmitter release, reduces inflammation, and increases resilience to stress. In addition, it promotes a sense of vigor and mental clarity. There are studies showing positive effects even on fatigue and depressive symptoms.

3. Dark room for sleep

Dark environments are essential for deep sleep. Use blackout curtains, eliminate device lights, and, if necessary, use a sleep mask. This supports natural melatonin production.

4. Absolute silence, or white noise

Avoid noise during the night. I like to use white noise to mask outside sounds. This helps achieve deeper sleep phases, such as REM sleep, and reduces nighttime awakenings.

5. Turn off electronics and Wi-Fi

Electromagnetic fields may interfere with the activity of the autonomic nervous system. Keep your phone away from the bed and on airplane mode. A good tip: turn off the Wi-Fi and step barefoot on the grass, a simple grounding practice.

6. Relax before sleeping

Avoid agitating movies, arguments, or excessive lighting. Create an atmosphere of calm. Diaphragmatic breathing techniques, soothing music, and light reading help prepare the brain for sleep. Give the body and mind time to slow down.

7. Go to sleep before midnight

Ideally, go to bed around 10:00 p.m. Melatonin peaks between 9:00 p.m. and 11:00 p.m. Sleeping during this window favors cellular regeneration and body recovery. Establish a fixed bedtime and wake-up time, this reinforces your circadian rhythm.

8. Avoid training at night

Intense physical activity after 4:00 p.m. may make the slowing-down process more difficult. If you are going to train at night, you will need to make a greater effort to relax afterward. Prefer lighter exercise during that period.

9. Move your body in the morning

Morning exercise releases endorphins and dopamine, reduces stress, increases productivity, and activates the brain. Even a simple morning cardio session can make a difference in your energy and mental clarity.

10. Avoid blue light at night

The blue light emitted by screens delays melatonin production. I use blue-light-blocking glasses to watch TV or use my phone. It is a simple and effective way to protect your sleep.

11. Caffeine only until 1:00 p.m.

Caffeine stays in the body for many hours and interferes with sleep depth. It blocks the receptors responsible for inducing sleep. Avoid coffee and stimulants in the afternoon.

12. No television in the bedroom, and have sex

The bedroom should be a space reserved for sleep, and sex. Even reading in the bedroom may confuse your brain and make sleep onset more difficult. Have separate environments for each activity.

After orgasm, a neuroendocrine response occurs that favors relaxation and the transition to sleep. There is an increase in prolactin, associated with satiety and sleepiness, and an increase in oxytocin, which reduces anxiety and activates the parasympathetic nervous system. At the same time, cortisol decreases, reducing alertness, and endorphins are released, promoting well-being and bodily relaxation.

13. Avoid heavy meals at night

Eating late and in large amounts overloads the digestive system and may cause reflux, impairing sleep. Have your last meal at least two hours before bed. The ideal? Dinner by 8:00 p.m., or even better, by 6:30 p.m.

14. Hydrate intelligently

Drink plenty of water throughout the day, but reduce intake at night to avoid bathroom trips during the night. Frequent interruptions compromise the body's restoration during sleep.

15. Create a sleep ritual

Establish a nighttime routine. A hot shower before bed, for example, causes peripheral vasodilation, which leads to heat loss and internal cooling of the body, this naturally increases melatonin production. This effect is scientifically proven.

The quality of your sleep does not depend only on the number of hours you sleep, but on the quality of your habits. Simple and conscious adjustments to your routine can profoundly transform your health, energy, and well-being. Choose some of these practices and start today, your body and mind will thank you.

Sleeping well is a revolutionary act in a world that idolizes cxhaustion. It is when we honor the body itself, restore the nervous system, clear away the excesses of the day, and allow the brain to rebuild itself for tomorrow.

Perhaps, in the end, true modern luxury is not having time, money, or power. It is lying down at night with a peaceful mind and waking up with a renewed body.

Putting It Into Practice:

- Start by implementing some of the sleep hygiene steps mentioned above. The important thing is to begin and turn it into a habit.
- Turn off screens 1 hour before bed and observe the impact on sleep quality.
- Try magnesium or meditation before bed and write down how you feel the next day.

CHAPTER 12

DOPAMINE DETOX: HOW TO REPROGRAM YOUR BRAIN

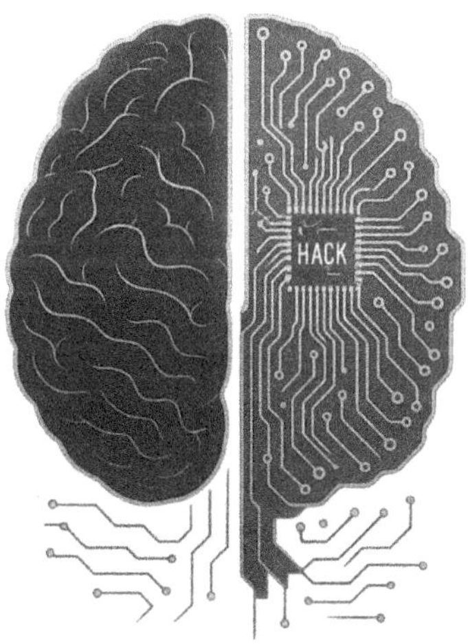

We live in the age of overstimulation. Every second, notifications compete for our attention, short videos hypnotize us, and likes, messages, and endless feeds flood the brain with small doses of pleasure. We are always "on," yet increasingly more unfocused, anxious, and exhausted.

This scenario has a clear neurochemical explanation: excess dopamine in disordered spikes. And that is affecting our motivation, our ability to focus, and even our sense of purpose.

Dopamine is a neurotransmitter involved in the anticipation of pleasure, motivation, and seeking behavior. Contrary to what many people think, it is not exactly the "pleasure hormone," but rather the messenger of desire, of wanting. It drives us to act toward something.

But in the modern environment, this system, which evolved to make us seek food, sex, and safety, has been hijacked by easy, constant digital stimuli.

Every click, like, short video, or notification activates the dopaminergic circuit, and the brain learns to seek more of it. This leads us into a cycle of compulsive novelty seeking, with less tolerance for boredom, deep concentration, and prolonged effort.

"We are living through a collective collapse of attention, and this is not a personal flaw, it is an environmental failure." Johann Hari, author of Stolen Focus.

When the brain gets used to instant and frequent rewards, such as those provided by social media, pornography, fast food, and digital games, it begins to lower its dopaminergic sensitivity.

That means less motivation for complex and slow activities, such as reading, studying, or long-term projects, less pleasure in natural and subtle experiences, and more apathy, procrastination, and compulsive seeking of distractions.

This dopaminergic desensitization is very similar to what happens in chemical addictions, such as alcohol or drugs: more stimulation is needed to feel the same pleasure.

Doing a "dopamine detox" does not mean eliminating this neurotransmitter, but rather reducing artificial stimuli and allowing the brain to regain its natural sensitivity. In other words, it means relearning how to feel pleasure from what is simple, calm, and real.

There are several strategies for reprogramming your brain. I can mention a few, for example: practice meditation and conscious breathing, because they train the brain to become less reactive and more present. They reduce the automatic impulse to seek stimulation every second.

Establish moments of the day without screens, especially in the first hour of the morning and the last hour before going to sleep. This time without artificial dopamine allows the brain to "breathe."

Keep a boredom and introspection journal. Writing down thoughts during moments of boredom can reveal creative insights and help you rediscover your inner voice. Boredom is fertile. It is there that the mind leaves consumption mode and enters creation mode.

Spend time in nature whenever you can. Walking, cooking, listening to music without distractions, playing with your children, contemplating the sky, all of this reactivates the genuine pleasure of lived experience, without the need for digital reward.

Practice delay gratification. Postpone rewards: study for 30 minutes before checking your phone, or leave social media for after completing a meaningful task. This retrains the dopaminergic circuit to work in favor of discipline.

To experience the power of a reset in practice, I propose the following exercise:

- Spend a full 24 hours without accessing social media, short videos, or digital entertainment content. During that period, write down how you feel: is there anxiety? Boredom? Clarity? Surprise? Also observe what arises in the silence: ideas, desires, memories.

This experiment is uncomfortable at first, but deeply revealing. It is like silencing a noisy band so you can finally hear your own heart.

Starting today, set a fixed daily time without screens, for example, the first hour of the day. When you wake up, no phone, email, or social media. Just you, your mind, and the real world. Open the curtain, the window, breathe deeply, receive the sunlight. This habit completely changes the way the day unfolds.

Dopamine detox is not about punishment, isolation, or being anti-technology. It is about reclaiming autonomy over your own mind. Instead of being pulled outward by stimuli, you begin directing your attention inward. It is learning to savor simplicity, revalue silence, and rediscover true motivation: the kind that does not come from likes, but from purpose.

"Attention is the foundation of all experience. When we lose attention, we lose everything." James Williams, former Google engineer and author of *Stand Out of Our Light*.

CHAPTER 13

HORMONAL REGULATION AND LONGEVITY

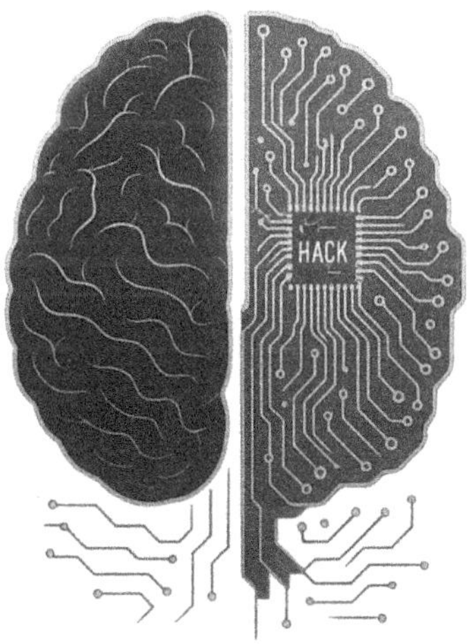

Talking about longevity without talking about hormones is like talking about an orchestra without mentioning the conductor. Hormones are the chemical messengers that organize the body's functioning: they regulate sleep, mood, metabolism, libido, strength, focus, and even the will to live.

Over time, these messengers can become imbalanced, whether because of age, chronic stress, poor diet, or a lifestyle disconnected from what is natural. But the good news is that hormones are modifiable. They respond to stimuli, habits, nutrients, and even to the way we think and move through the world.

Among the hormones with the greatest impact on vitality and longevity are: testosterone, responsible for energy, libido, cognition, muscle strength, and motivation; progesterone, which helps with sleep, stress regulation, and nervous system balance; GH, growth hormone, which supports cellular regeneration, muscle tone, and body composition; and cortisol, which drives the stress response, morning energy, and metabolism.

When these substances are in harmony, the body functions with power and ease. But when they are dysregulated, everything seems harder, from sleep to libido, from concentration to the immune system.

The secret of hormonal modulation is not synthetic hormones as a first-line approach, but rather the creation of a favorable physiological environment in which the body returns to producing and responding properly to its own messengers.

Let us see how these hormones work.

Testosterone is much more than a sex hormone, it is a marker of vitality. Adequate levels are associated with more lean mass, better cognition, stable mood, and lower risk of metabolic disease. Some practical strategies help increase testosterone naturally:

- Deep and consistent sleep, 7.5 to 9 hours per night.
- Strength training and compound exercises, squats, deadlifts, and so on.
- Controlled intermittent fasting, respecting body type and context.
- Morning sun exposure, which regulates the circadian cycle and improves hormone production.
- Zinc, vitamin D, magnesium, and boron are cofactors for testosterone synthesis.
- Reducing plastics, pesticides, and endocrine disruptors, such as BPA and phthalates.
- Avoiding chronic cortisol spikes, which inhibit testosterone.

"Lifestyle shapes more hormones than any pharmacy formula." Dr. Andrew Huberman, neuroscientist at Stanford University.

Progesterone acts as women's natural calming hormone, helping regulate sleep, mood, and anxiety. After age 35, its production tends to decline, especially in anovulatory cycles or in situations of chronic stress.

Natural ways to stimulate progesterone:

- Stress and cortisol management, chronically high cortisol "steals" progesterone.

- Consumption of healthy fats, avocado, olive oil, seeds, omega-3.
- Vitamins B6, C, and E, essential for the synthesis of this hormone.
- Maca root and vitex agnus-castus, chasteberry, are herbal remedies with gentle regulatory action.

GH is released mainly during deep sleep and after high-intensity exercise. It helps tissue regeneration, increases lean mass, and promotes fat burning. How can it be naturally stimulated?

- With fasted training that includes explosive muscular effort, HIIT or sprints.
- By practicing an overnight fast of at least 12 hours.
- By avoiding sugar at night, since insulin inhibits GH release.
- By sleeping before 11:00 p.m., since GH peaks early in the night.

And then we have cortisol, which is essential, because it is what wakes us up in the morning, regulates blood sugar, and helps us respond to challenges.

But the problem is chronic excess, which leads to exhaustion, anxiety, catabolism, and lowered immunity.

Some changes in routine help modulate cortisol, such as exposure to natural light in the morning and reduced blue light at night, avoiding caffeine after 2:00 p.m., practicing deep nasal breathing, yoga, meditation, and walking outdoors. Using adaptogens such as ashwagandha, rhodiola, and eleuthero helps the body cope better with stress.

The endocrine system is like an orchestra: complex, interdependent, and sensitive to any discord. Each hormone acts like an instrument that must come in at the right moment, in the right dose, to ensure the body's harmony. And that is exactly where medicinal plants and bioactive nutrients come into play, not as artificial hormone substitutes, but as natural tuners, capable of regulating this internal symphony with precision and gentleness.

Unlike hormone replacement therapies, which often impose a forced rhythm on the body and may bring side effects, phytonutrients and adaptogens have the capacity to modulate the functioning of the hormonal axis intelligently. They do not force the body to produce more or less, but help restore lost balance.

Among the most studied adaptogens, ashwagandha stands out for its action on the hypothalamic-pituitary-adrenal, HPA, axis, reducing cortisol levels, the main stress hormone, while at the same time promoting an increase in testosterone in both men and women, as demonstrated by various clinical studies. Rhodiola rosea is known for its ability to increase mental focus and resistance to physical and emotional stress, making it especially useful in times of exhaustion.

For women, maca root offers remarkable benefits for mood, libido, and hormonal balance throughout the cycle and menopause. And tribulus terrestris, although it has a more modest effect on testosterone, may be useful in cases of low libido or low vitality.

Beyond plants, certain nutrients play a fundamental role in maintaining hormonal health. Vitamin D3 combined with K2 acts as a hormonal signaler, positively influencing various systems in the body, including the immune and reproductive systems. Magnesium, especially in the threonate and glycinate forms, contributes to the regulation of sleep, mood, and the HPA axis. Zinc is essential for testosterone production and thyroid function, while folate and vitamin B12 are indispensable for methylation and hormonal detoxification processes, processes that, when inefficient, can lead to the buildup of inflammatory hormonal metabolites.

Maintaining a regular exercise routine, especially strength training, is one of the most effective strategies for preserving hormonal production, especially testosterone, GH, and insulin. An anti-inflammatory diet, rich in whole foods, vegetables, and essential micronutrients, offers the metabolic support necessary for proper hormone synthesis and metabolism.

Another critical factor is exposure to environmental toxins. Compounds such as bisphenol A, found in plastics, pesticides, solvents, and heavy metals are known endocrine disruptors, meaning they directly interfere with hormone production and action. Avoiding excessive contact with these substances is a powerful way to protect the endocrine system throughout life.

Preserving the health of the HPA axis, responsible for coordinating the stress response, is equally fundamental. And that is not done only with supplements or calming teas, but with consistent practices: quality sleep, contact with nature, intentional breaks during the day, and a less overstimulated life. An exhausted HPA axis leads to cascading dysfunction, from the thyroid to the adrenals, from sex hormones to immunity.

Finally, insulin and blood sugar control must be a priority. Excess insulin in the blood, very common in diets rich in refined carbohydrates and poor in fiber, accelerates the aging of the hormonal system, favoring conditions such as leptin resistance, abdominal obesity, inflammation, and chronic fatigue.

In short, hormonal longevity does not depend on magic formulas, but on a well-tuned orchestra made of conscious choices, healthy habits, and the careful use of plants and nutrients that respect the body's intelligence. It is possible to age with vitality, libido, mental clarity, and energy, provided the hormonal symphony is conducted wisely.

The key to longevity is not just living longer, but living with vitality, desire, mental clarity, and energy. And hormones are the messengers of that internal state. The human body has an incredible capacity to rebalance itself when the soil is fertile.

You do not need to wait for symptoms to appear or for lab work to be "outside the reference range." With awareness, information, and small daily practices, it is possible to modulate aging and expand life with power and presence.

The human body is highly sensitive to the environment in which it lives. Each small choice throughout the day, the light that enters the eyes at dawn, the foods consumed, the type of movement performed, or the time spent under stress, profoundly shapes the hormonal system. That is why a routine aligned with biological rhythms is the best "supplement" that exists. As I have said before, having a healthy routine is everything.

A hormonally healthy day begins as soon as you wake up. Exposing the eyes to sunlight within the first 30 minutes of the day is one of the most powerful habits for synchronizing the circadian cycle and stimulating natural morning cortisol production, which will bring focus, energy, and mood regulation throughout the day. It is the first step toward a balanced hormonal axis.

Moving the body in the morning, even with a simple walk or stretching, already activates testosterone and GH. And a well-built breakfast, with protein, healthy fats, and few sugars, ensures steady energy without the spikes and crashes typical of an inflammatory diet.

In the afternoon, it is worth reinforcing nutrition with varied vegetables, micronutrients such as zinc and magnesium, and, if necessary, vitamin D supplementation, ideally accompanied by vitamin K2 to optimize its action. A brief pause in the middle of the day, with conscious breathing or meditation, helps modulate cortisol and prevents its chronic buildup, a major saboteur of hormonal balance.

At night, everything changes. The body needs signals of slowing down to understand that it is time to produce melatonin and regenerate. Reducing bright lights, avoiding screen use after 9:00 p.m., and respecting a fixed bedtime, preferably before 11:00 p.m., are habits just as important as any supplement.

It is during these moments of deep rest that the rejuvenation hormones come into play: GH, melatonin, and progesterone work silently to repair tissues, strengthen the mind, and preserve vitality.

The proposal here is not to wait until disease appears in order to treat it, but to cultivate an internal environment in which disease does not thrive. That is true preventive medicine, a model of life in which hormones work in our favor, as allies of vitality.

Instead of trying to fix imbalances with immediate external solutions, it is wiser to ask: what is dysregulating my internal orchestra? The answer will almost always be in the details of your routine, in the quality of your sleep, in the nature of your diet, in the type of stress you carry, and in how you deal with it.

Modulating hormones is, ultimately, learning to live better, with presence, clarity, and strength, throughout all the cycles of life.

Task:

- Have you noticed signs of hormonal imbalance in your daily life? For example: fatigue, irritability, poor sleep? Write them down and observe patterns in your lifestyle.
- If possible, get hormone testing done and record the results for future comparisons.

BONUS CHAPTERS

CHAPTER 14

MEDICINE AND SPIRITUALITY, HEALING THAT TRANSCENDS THE BODY

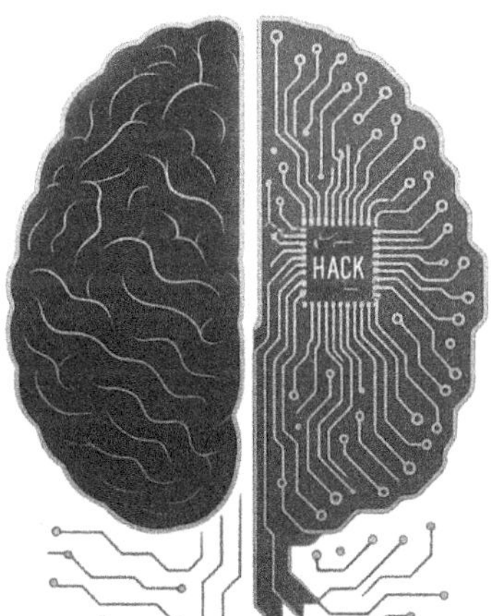

Writing these pages is a gift. They are born from a real story, lived with affection, purpose, and truth. A story that began more than a decade ago, when life asked for my full presence and revealed to me, in practice, that body, mind, and spirit form a sacred unity.

It was shortly after the birth of my second son, Pedro. We went through delicate days in the ICU. As a mother, I remained in vigil, sustained by faith. My soul was steady, spirituality pulsed within me with clarity, but I knew I needed to care for my physical body so that it would be equal to the strength of my spirit. I had always believed that life is vibration. And, in order to sustain that vibration with strength, I decided to realign my body, strengthen my system, and give it the support the mission required.

That was how I met Dr. José Roberto, Beto. It was not just an appointment, it was a meeting of destiny. I entered his office seeking balance for the body and found a partnership of souls. Beto cared for me with scientific precision and human sensitivity. He adjusted hormones, monitored lab tests, and reorganized my metabolism. But there was something beyond the medical protocol. A vibrational affinity blossomed, and with it came the certainty that health is not merely the absence of disease, but coherence among body, mind, emotions, and spirit.

Our appointments became profound dialogues. He brought the rigor of medicine, and I brought the language of energy, vibration, and active faith. We discovered that true transformation was born from that synergy. Beto began to observe carefully the way I spoke about energy and God, and I shared my cellular and atomic understanding of spirituality. I explained how every thought generates electrical discharges in the brain, how every feeling modulates the magnetic field of the heart, and how, when both align, coherence arises. And coherence reorganizes the nervous system, instructs the cells, and favors healing.

I had always lived that within myself. My daily prayers and meditations helped me maintain vibrant health. I spoke to my cells as someone honoring a team of light working in my favor. He saw this reflected in my consistent lab results, and our friendship also became a study partnership. Over time, we began helping people together: he with medicine as a divine tool, and I with spirituality as a force of vibrational support.

One experience in particular left its mark on me. Beto invited me to accompany an elderly woman in the terminal phase of life. She had hurt many people throughout her life and now feared death. Her body no longer responded, but her soul was still crying out for help. I sat beside her and spoke about the power of forgiveness, explaining that forgiveness does not set only the other person free, but also oneself. At first, she resisted. Pride seemed greater than her own pain. But something in her opened. Little by little, she sought out those she had hurt, asked for forgiveness from the heart, and was forgiven. Not long afterward, she passed away in peace. There was no healing of the body, but there was liberation of the soul. There I understood, once again, that healing is always expansion.

That experience, and so many others, solidified our shared mission. Science and spirituality do not compete, they complement one another. And since then, I have been certain that everything in life is vibration, and that the vibration we sustain shapes our reality.

Vibration is the essence of everything. Nothing in the universe is static: everything pulses at specific frequencies. So do we. Every thought we generate produces electrical activity in the brain. Every feeling we nurture creates a magnetic field that emanates from the heart. Together, they form our personal electromagnetic field, our vibrational signature. When that field is misaligned, the body becomes fragile. When mind and heart unite in coherence, the field grows stronger and the body finds pathways to balance.

Neuroscience confirms what spirituality has always known. The practice of gratitude, for example, strengthens areas of the brain linked to emotional regulation, releases dopamine and serotonin, and reduces inflammatory processes. Love expands the heart's electromagnetic field up to five thousand times more than the brain's field, influencing not only the one who feels it, but everyone around. To love and to give thanks are not merely spiritual gestures: they are scientific practices of health.

I also speak of manifestation. To manifest is not to wish superficially, but to sustain an inner state compatible with what one wishes to live. To manifest vitality, healing, and balance, a strong vibrational field is necessary. Clear thoughts and elevated feelings join together to form electromagnetic waves capable of reorganizing cells and reprogramming patterns. Biology responds to vibration.

For more than a decade alongside Beto, I observed the same phenomenon in many patients: people with an elevated vibrational field show faster and more effective cellular recovery. They heal better, respond with greater quality to treatments, and reorganize systems more easily. This realization showed us that the medicine of the future is preventive, and vibrational prevention is its pillar.

Biohacking, often seen only as technology or supplementation, is also a path of vibrational prevention. Every physical choice reverberates in the energetic field. Foods are not only nutrients, they are living frequencies. Herbs and teas carry subtle forces that dialogue with our cells and with the soul. Fasting reorganizes metabolism, but it also expands mental clarity. Physical movement does not only strengthen muscles, it awakens vital energy. Deep sleep regenerates the body and purifies the vibrational field. The sun adjusts internal rhythms and awakens the memory that we are part of the whole. Contact with the earth, water, and forests grounds and harmonizes us. Conscious breathing and presence restore coherence. Every simple practice is, in truth, vibrational medicine.

And there is still a higher key: virtues. Love, gratitude, faith, compassion, joy, and courage are not merely human values, but living frequencies that transform our biology and elevate our consciousness. When we tune ourselves to these virtues, our vibrational framework reorganizes. Gratitude strengthens neural networks of belonging, activates well-being hormones, and reinforces immunity. Love reorganizes physiology and expands the cardiac field. Compassion opens space for cellular and emotional repair.

When we are vibrationally strong, self-care ceases to be an effort and becomes natural. Meditation becomes pleasure. Prayer becomes breath. Eating well becomes an act of love. Exercising becomes awakening energy. Being with family, with a spouse and children, becomes nourishment for the soul. True friendships, hobbies, and new learning cease to be distractions and become practices of vibrational nourishment. We recognize who we are: precious beings. And we begin to use time in our favor.

I carry in my heart stories that prove this truth. Women who tried to become pregnant for years and who, by uniting Beto's medical treatments with the spiritual strengthening I guided, now hold children in their arms. People who arrived fragile and rediscovered vitality because they learned to vibrate in love and gratitude. Patients who, after understanding the vibrational field, regained physical, mental, and emotional health.

It is an honor to have Beto in my life. Our friendship is made of trust, respect, and admiration. We share paths, studies, and experiences that help us grow together. And we have lived unforgettable moments side by side. One of them will remain forever marked in me: I had the joy of officiating his wedding to Priscila. It was moving to witness that love, to unite two souls before life, and to see a new family begin. There, we were not merely doctor and patient, but soul friends. There, entire families were present, embracing each other in partnership and affection. This friendship is also a family partnership, one that grows stronger every day and inspires us to help all the people who cross our path.

Being part of this book is yet another honor. It translates the mission we share: science and spirituality united in favor of life.

Everything in life is vibration. The vibration we sustain with thoughts and feelings shapes our reality. When we believe in our divine potential, we find the key to true healing. Our body is our instrument of divine work. It is through it that the soul manifests, consciousness expands, and the mission is fulfilled. We are here to evolve spiritually. Caring for the physical body, the mind, the emotions, and the spirit is the path to that evolution. And at the center of everything there is only one frequency: love. Love is the highest force, the most powerful healing, the energy that sustains life.

Remember: LOVE is, and always will be, the key to everything!

With love and gratitude,

Lu Matosinhos

Speaker, Vibrational Mentor, and Neuroscientist

specialized in Spirituality.

CHAPTER 15

CONSISTENCY, THE BEHAVIORS BEHIND EVERY TRANSFORMATION

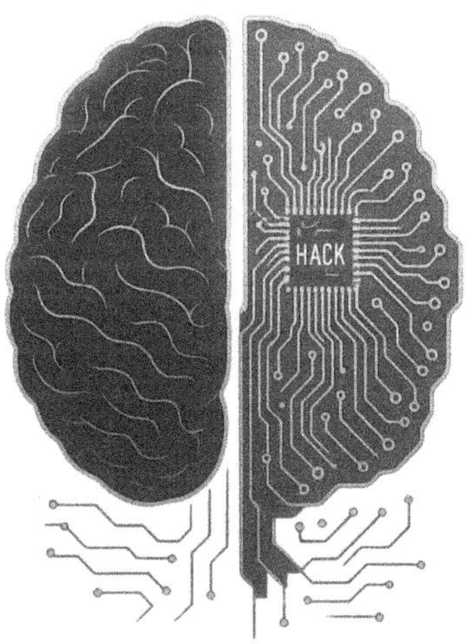

The best programs will never work for you until you have a disciplined enough mind to follow them. Spartan warriors were known for having a mindset that dealt with the problems that arose by being devoted to rigorous training and to the "religion" of physical culture. You can learn to think like the "300" as well.

"Spartans never retreat, Spartans never surrender. Let every Greek come to know this truth, let each of them seek it within himself. No retreat and no surrender. This is the law of Sparta. And by the law of Sparta we shall fight, fight and die. Honor those shields, warriors! Au!"

After doing that, you will be at least halfway to having the body of your dreams. When it comes to thinking like a proud member of the "300," remember these things:

Think positive

The mind can either drain you or motivate you when you face challenges. Getting in shape is certainly a difficult challenge for most people. Adopting the habit of thinking and speaking positively can change your game.

Clear your mind of negative self-talk and immediately replace it with messages like "It is challenging, but I can do it." Notice how much more power that will give you to get things done instantly!

Be prepared for sacrifice

Nothing exceptionally good happens without hard work. That is an unavoidable truth, despite what the gurus out there may try to sell.

If you want to be everything you were born to be, you must be prepared to work hard. Sculpting a new you is not easy, but all your sweat, time, and hard work will be worth it. Trust me.

Write down your goals

Spartans set goals and achieve them, so put on paper everything you want to accomplish. Whenever you feel like quitting, look at your goals and renew your energy. Dedicating a few minutes a day to writing down your daily goals and half an hour or more on the weekend to outlining weekly and monthly goals can be the difference between succeeding and failing in your program.

All warriors set goals

Historical studies have shown that Spartan leaders were obsessive about planning, far more than any other leader of their time. When you set a goal, it becomes much easier to achieve it!

The will to act

This is the most important Spartan mental trait you must adopt if you want to sculpt your warrior physique. Embracing this mindset will make achieving anything much easier.

It is what 95% of people in the world lack: the will to act. You can have all the knowledge in the world and the best intentions, but if you do not act on them, the chances of change in your life are reduced to almost nothing. Act quickly and consistently and, at the very least, you will have a chance to see your life improve. Sitting around and feeling sorry for yourself will get you nowhere.

Training methods and winning attitudes that worked in the past still work today. We are still the same human beings with the same physical makeup, and we respond in the same way to adversity.

You need patience

Are you patient enough to achieve the body you want? Patience is a highly underestimated virtue and is of the utmost importance when it comes to transforming your body and restoring your health. Christian author Joyce Meyer once said:

"Patience is not the ability to wait, but the ability to keep a good attitude while waiting."

There is tremendous wisdom in this quote, and it is something every person should remember when striving for a worthy goal, especially those trying to lose weight and get in shape, for example.

If you are trying to lose weight, it will take time. An average person can only lose about 2 kilograms of fat per week. If you are 30 kilograms overweight, that will equal about 15 weeks, which is almost 4 months. Many enthusiastic people make New Year's resolutions to lose weight and believe it will all be over by the end of January. They do not even realize it may take until the end of April to reach their goals.

If your weight-loss progress plateaus, which is very common, it will take even longer to reach your ideal weight. The goal may only come true in June, for example. Half the year will already be gone, do you have the patience to wait that long?

How motivated are you to exercise? How happy are you? These next steps may help you.

Practice gratitude

You will feel much more positive and ready to deal with any situation when you can feel gratitude every day. Consider creating a gratitude habit in which you write down or say to yourself a few things you are grateful for every day. You can do this before going to bed at night or first thing in the morning.

Meditate

Meditation reduces stress and increases happiness. You do not have to meditate for hours to reap the benefits. Start with just a few minutes a day. There are apps, podcasts, YouTube channels, and online tools you can use to help establish a practice.

Take a cold shower when you wake up

A cold shower improves blood circulation, helps stimulate the immune system, speeds up metabolism, helps relieve pain and recover muscles, and is excellent for skin health. Cold showers help by training your nervous system to be more resistant to stress and adversity. Some studies have pointed out that this habit acts as a small oxidative form of stress on your nervous system, and over time your body adapts to it.

Take a hot shower before bed

Want to establish a relaxing routine to sleep better? Take a hot shower. It lowers your heart rate and calms your mind and body so you can fall asleep easily.

Spend time in nature

Get 15 to 20 minutes of sun exposure per day. This will help your body produce vitamin D. It also improves mood and reduces stress. Go outside every day, even if it is just for a short walk.

Practice grounding

Grounding is the name given to the practice that allows us to have direct and transformative contact with Mother Earth. Practicing grounding regularly can reduce symptoms such as anxiety, depression, and others that directly affect our lives. That is why there has been so much discussion about the importance of walking barefoot on the ground or grass.

There are simple steps you can take every day to improve your overall health and well-being. We are talking about moving more, reducing stress, and sleeping better. Your daily habits make all the difference.

Stressed? Walk it off

Instead of eating, shopping, or giving in to a television binge, go for a walk when you are stressed. It is better for your health and will truly change your mindset. You will relax and feel lighter.

Use a standing desk

Speaking of moving your body, if you sit all day, consider getting a standing desk. It does not have to be complicated. You do not need to build or buy anything. In many cases, you can simply stack boxes on your desk, place your computer on them, and stand for a while. You will improve your health and fitness. People who sit most of the day are 54% more likely to die from a heart attack.

Turn off snooze mode

Struggle to get up in the morning? Put your phone far away from your bed, preferably in another room, get up immediately after hearing it ring, wash your face right away, and make your bed. That will drastically reduce the chances of your lying down again. You can complete your morning routine with a gratitude habit, meditation, and a cold shower.

If you lose to a simple alarm clock, what can you actually win against?

Sleep more

Sleep has been proven to help with weight loss and reduce the risk of obesity. It is also essential for post-workout recovery. To improve your health at every level, make sure you are sleeping enough. What is enough? In general, 7 to 8 hours. Implement systems to gradually improve the quality and quantity of your sleep. For example, you can put your phone on airplane mode starting at 8:00 p.m. and avoid using any electronics after that time.

Give up alcohol

Alcohol disrupts sleep and reduces its quality. It also stresses your systems so your body cannot repair and renew itself, and it dehydrates you. Take a look at how often you drink and set a goal to stop. When you do drink, prefer wine. Remember to drink plenty of water.

Stop smoking "USB sticks"

Stop smoking any kind of cigarette, including marijuana. It may seem cool to your friends, but believe me, you are getting nothing good from adopting this habit. On the contrary, in the long run it will ruin your health. Be a Spartan and do not put that garbage in your mouth.

Adopting this Spartan mindset will eliminate weakness from your life.

Are you ready to join the "300"?

Then get up and start working hard today!

Forget motivation

One of the hardest parts of any training program is the motivation to keep going. However, it is easier to stay motivated if you are a weightlifter. That is because you can see and feel the results in a short time. Lift weights for just a few weeks and you will begin to see a 20 to 40% increase in your strength and endurance almost immediately. And it will not just be during your workout sessions. Suddenly all those grocery bags you carry home will feel much lighter. More strength and power will improve any sport you choose to practice. Stronger leg muscles will allow you to run faster. A stronger upper body will allow you to throw any object farther. Weightlifting and strength training improve overall conditioning, and stronger muscles and bones can take more impact, so lifting weights can help prevent sports-related injuries.

But after all, what is more important in my fitness journey, motivation or discipline?

This is an excellent question, and there is only one answer, discipline. To be more specific, you need self-discipline to achieve anything worthwhile in fitness and in life.

So what is the difference between the two?

When New Year's is approaching, feeling excited and motivated to make big life changes is very common. That is an example of motivation from external sources.

Every year, millions of people make resolutions to lose weight, get in shape, save money, and so on. They are inspired and motivated by the date. New Year's feels like a fresh start. Everything seems possible.

However, by February, millions of people give up on their resolutions and the year seems as though it will be like any other, at least until the next New Year's, when the cycle repeats.

So why do they give up? The bitter truth is that if someone does what they have always done, they will stay where they have always been. To see new results and achieve high goals, you will need to make major changes in your life. Unfortunately, almost all change is met with opposition.

Trying to clean up your diet and lose weight? You will have to get used to the new nutritious foods you need to eat. You will need to stop watching so much TV and go to the gym and train.

These new changes will seem unbearable and unpleasant. Nutritious foods will seem bland to you. You will crave junk food and sugary, processed foods. You will have to fight those temptations constantly, and that is not fun. Therefore, you need self-discipline to stay on track, a lot of self-discipline. If you lack it, you will give in to temptation.

As Steven Covey said:

"The undisciplined are slaves to moods, appetites and passions."

Develop self-discipline

Once the promise of a new beginning and the festive spirit of New Year's are over, that is when routine sets in and motivation can die very quickly. In times like these, discipline will take you where motivation cannot. It is essential that you develop self-discipline. That is the key to achieving all the goals you have always wanted. It is a skill that makes you almost unstoppable. You can watch all the self-help videos and motivational talks on the planet. You can work yourself into a frenzy of motivation all night, but when morning comes and you need to wake up early to go run, and you do not do it, all that motivation will have been for nothing. If you had self-discipline, you would grimace and get up. You may not like it, but you will do it, and when you finish, you will have the satisfaction of knowing you kept your promises to yourself. Self-discipline will make you respect yourself and grow as a person. You will begin to become the person others look to for motivation. Your fitness levels will skyrocket through consistent effort, and your body will transform into a machine. Not through motivation, but through discipline.

"Motivation gets you started, discipline keeps you going."

Evolve so much that others will need to get to know you again

Analyze your progress objectively. Any long journey requires a map to make sure you reach your destination correctly. Even airplanes that fly at such high altitudes require pilots to make many course corrections to guide them to their destination. Even when there are no obstacles, it is easy for a plane to drift off course.

It is worth remembering this analogy when you make a New Year's resolution to get fit and healthy. In theory, you only need to eat less and exercise more.

There is a saying that goes:

"In theory, theory and practice are the same. In practice, they are not."

You will discover this when you actually try to cut out junk food and eat clean. Suddenly, you will have cravings and will constantly be thinking about food throughout the day. You did not expect it to be so hard, but it is.

Your workout sessions, which were supposed to be a breeze, turn into a grind. You had no idea it would be so exhausting, but it is. So what do most people do? They quit, and once they do, their goals are over.

The key to progressing and staying on track until you reach your fitness goals will be analyzing your progress once a week. That is the best way to stay focused and make sure you do not drift off course.

Analyzing your progress

The first thing you will need to do is take pictures to analyze the before and after. Every week, you will need an action plan to eat well, and you will need to know how often you are going to the gym and what you will be doing there. Be an organized person, you should have everything written down to make it easy to refer back to. Your goal will be to stick to this plan as best you can. Every day you will check where you followed the plan and where you failed. It is inevitable to slip here and there, but do your best to stay on track and achieve at least an 80% success rate.

Looking for improvements

At the end of each week, look at where you did well and where you slipped. See whether you notice any patterns. You may discover that every time you have a social night with friends, you abandon your diet and eat uncontrollably. You will need to avoid all social events until you have made considerable progress in your fitness journey and are able not to be influenced by the environment. It will be easier to stay on track when you have developed more self-discipline. In addition to just sticking to the plan, try to find ways to improve your performance. There is always room for improvement.

You may try lifting more weight at the gym or improving your sprints by a few seconds. You may do an extra mobility workout on Wednesdays and Sundays. There are many ways to improve, write down what you need to do and do your best to carry it out. Check whether you are making progress. If you are, wonderful. If not, do not get discouraged.

Remember this phrase from Joel Jota, former Brazilian National Swimming Team athlete, whenever you think about quitting:

"They will get tired, most people do, most people are undisciplined. You do not fail to achieve things because you lack knowledge, but because you lack discipline."

Therefore, look at your notes and try to figure out where you may have slipped. Do you need to watch your calories more closely? Do you need to train with greater intensity? Sometimes your body needs time to adapt and you will only see improvements after two weeks or more. What matters is that you analyze your actions daily, stay on track, and monitor your overall progress once a week. That is the best way to succeed in the long term.

"Things work out best for those who make the best of how things work out." John Wooden

There is no perfection

Perfectionism has ruined more goals and dreams than you can imagine. When New Year's approaches, millions of people make serious resolutions to get fit and healthy. They want their efforts to be perfect, but they make the fatal mistake of ignoring the fact that no one is infallible and we all live in an imperfect world.

Salvador Dalí once said:

"Have no fear of perfection, you will never reach it."

Here is a very common scenario that repeats itself millions of times every year, and it is amazing that people still do it.

Let us say someone decides to clean up their diet and avoid all junk food. The first mistake is that people generally make changes that are too radical. They believe they can get results overnight through sheer willpower. The goal is to be perfect with their diet so that their new year will be clean and perfect.

Within a day or two, they realize how difficult it is to keep their diet super clean. Their hormones crave junk food all the time. Resisting becomes harder and harder, until finally they are exhausted and give in to temptation.

Within minutes, their ideal of perfection collapses on top of them. They failed.

When confronted with failure, they realize how far they are from what they believed they could achieve. The end result is that they feel guilty, useless, and think they lack discipline.

In reality, they were doomed to fail the moment they expected a perfect outcome. Life simply does not work that way.

The first step is to understand that you cannot build Rome in a day. You cannot transform your health and body immediately. You are fighting against years of bad habits. Your goal should be to make small positive changes every day that will translate into massive improvements in the long run.

If you eat 4 slices of pizza, cut it down to 2 slices. That is an improvement. It may not seem like much, but it will make all the difference over time.

The same applies to any junk food or processed foods. Eat them, but cut the portions in half. Doing that will reduce your calories and suffocate urges and cravings, because you are still giving your body what it wants. Little by little, day by day, you can free yourself from sugar addiction and replace junk food with healthier foods.

Does this process seem slow and imperfect? You bet it does. However, it is easier to follow through with it and stay on track. Your goal is to achieve small successes repeatedly. Those will be the inches you gain as you crawl toward the finish line. Do not use perfectionism as a crutch to criticize yourself or procrastinate. Instead, make a sensible action plan and pursue small daily improvements that will lead you to surprising long-term results. That is the best way to do it.

Luis Henrique Soares de Melo

Businessman, salesman, and sports enthusiast

CHAPTER 16

FUNCTIONAL NUTRITION, A TOOL FOR DIAGNOSIS AND HEALING

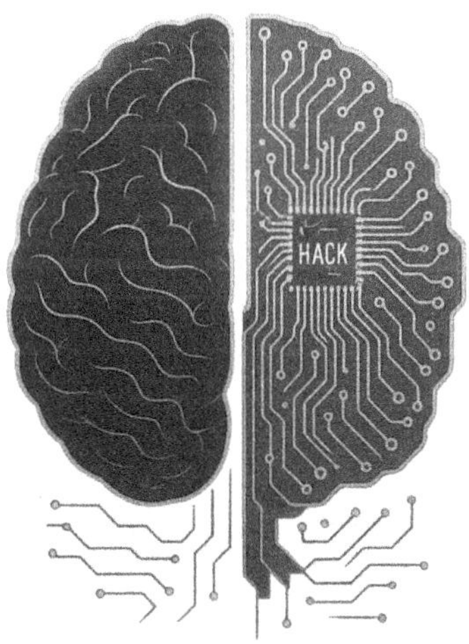

Humanity is constantly searching for the invention of the magic pill. The one that will solve every problem: weight loss, perfect skin, the necessary energy, a sound mind, and eternal life. The way things are going, I would not doubt that some genius will create shortcuts for that. But let the truth be told: WE ALREADY HAVE EVERYTHING IN OUR HANDS, yet it requires effort and sacrifice, which most people are not willing to pay the price for.

It may sound cliché to talk about food. Everyone has already heard Hippocrates' famous phrase: "*Let food be thy medicine and medicine be thy food.*" But it is impossible to keep talking about the steps of a biohacker without talking about our fuel. It is impossible to optimize human biology without fertile ground that receives good substrates.

Let us begin by thinking about how much food actually matters in our lives. What we see is the outside, but inside there is a very complex organism. There is an extensive digestive system and several stages of absorption and cellular nourishment. Just because you do not see it does not mean it is not happening. Most diseases began at some point long before the individual could notice them. You know that car that broke down on the road "out of nowhere"? We are just machines in constant use, and we need care so that we can remain functional for a long time.

That is why I separated out 3 tips that I consider the main topics of dietary care when it comes to preparing the body to live longer and better. And the first is the famous H2O, that is right.

If that is news to you, I do not know, but believe it: an average of 70% of our body is made up of WATER!

I know you imagined I would begin by asking you to consume imported foods with difficult names, but the basics need to be done. If we are basically water, why do we not worry about the water we drink? In fact, many people do not even drink water at all!

According to IPSEMG, the recommended daily intake is 35 ml of water for each kilogram of body weight. In other words, a person who weighs 80 kg x 35 ml needs to consume an average of 2.8 liters daily.

After understanding the minimum necessary amount, it is also necessary to consider quality. This matters because simply drinking water does not guarantee proper hydration capable of supplying our cells with the fluid they need to maintain their volume and perform their functions correctly.

There needs to be an exchange of water between the inside and outside of the cell, measured by the balance of solutes and water. That is why drinking too much water, or not drinking the minimum amount, and or not having the necessary electrolytes for that exchange, means nothing happens.

A classic example: have you noticed that whenever we get sick, whether from diarrhea or vomiting, and need to intensify hydration, the doctor always recommends homemade oral rehydration solution? Coconut water or other liquids with electrolyte-replacement effects? And have you ever stopped to think about the main composition of those solutions? I will tell you: water, sugar, and salt.

Glucose and sodium are absorbed by the intestine through the sodium-glucose system, which facilitates hydration of the cells. Of course, there are other important electrolytes in this process, such as the mineral potassium. But I wanted to illustrate this whole situation so you can connect it to what I am trying to tell you. So the trend of "water with unrefined salt" is not nonsense, it really does have some foundation. What happens is that the general population lives on foods that are extremely rich in sodium and sugar and does not drink water. But for an individual eating a natural diet, making a homemade solution with 1 liter of water and 1 coffee spoon, 3 g, of unrefined salt per day will be very welcome. The result of proper hydration is better concentration, agility, energy, youthful skin, strong hair and nails, and much more.

After understanding the quantity and the correct process of delivering water to our cells, it is worth questioning the type of water we are consuming, the same water that makes up 70% of our body. What we have is the famous "treated water," full of toxic metals and acidity. Nowadays it is possible to find filters with 3 candles that are able to remove a large part of these compounds, as well as filters with the ability to regulate the pH of the water.

And no, I am not saying that alkaline water alkalinizes the blood, because we have an ideal pH for that. But considering that even vegetables with pesticides already tend to be more acidic, one way to balance our diet, seeking a more alkaline environment that is less favorable to the emergence of disease, is to invest in good water.

After understanding hydration, a second point of dietary care is the adequate consumption of protein throughout the day. Since I like to paint a mental picture of how things work, imagine a pearl necklace. That necklace is a protein molecule in which each of those pearls represents an amino acid, in other words, a protein is formed by a set of amino acids. And for each specific combination, there is a different protein.

These amino acids are nutrients with diverse functions in our body, important for brain, cellular, and bone development, with a structural function in strengthening muscle tissues, maintaining bodily activities, and supporting the immune system.

When we talk about aging with quality, or better yet, being a functional older adult, one of the main points is the correct intake of protein combined with strengthening activities. Like bricks, these amino acids build our whole body. They participate in the production of hormones and neurotransmitters, make up membranes, contribute to the defense field of our antibodies, support muscle gain, and strengthen bones.

According to the WHO, World Health Organization, the recommendation is 0.8 grams of protein for each kilogram of body weight per day. Example: an individual weighing 80 kg x 0.8 g = 64 g. For those who practice physical activity, between 1.2 and 2.0 g per kg per day. In my clinical practice, I have always found the minimum recommendation low. I have always maintained values of 1.6 to 2.2 g per kg according to the activities of the day. It is worth remembering that the quantity in grams does not refer to the amount of food, but to the protein itself. As an example, a 100 g chicken breast has approximately 25 g of protein.

Nowadays it has become easier to look up the macronutrients of a food. The reference base in nutrition is the Taco Table, available in a free PDF online. But consulting that table through Artificial Intelligence, AI, is already a starting point. It is only important to emphasize that animal proteins are complete in amino acid diversity, while plant proteins require combinations.

Finally, and no less important, in the third topic I want to bring up the importance of proper antioxidant intake. After all, we live in a world where we are constantly being contaminated. Yes, that is exactly what you just read. It is air pollution, parasites surrounding us, foods, even natural ones, full of additives, skincare and cosmetic products with endocrine disruptors, plastic containers with toxic compounds, an extensive vaccine schedule, and so on.

But then a question remains: *is not our liver the organ responsible for our detoxification process?* True. But as much as over the years our body adapts to situations we expose it to, the truth is that the overload has been too much. And let us be honest, disease has never been talked about so much, even rare diseases that are now common, children with cancer, a disease that until then had been seen as a disease of older people.

Think of it this way: the point is not to shield ourselves from "bad things," because we do not live in a bubble. Of course, avoiding them is already a big step, and having good resources is too, which is exactly what this book teaches you. But beyond that, one way to neutralize the body's systemic inflammation is by delivering the necessary antioxidants, which are basically substances that help protect cells against damage caused by excess free radicals.

These free radicals are naturally produced by our body during metabolism and in response to external factors. In low amounts, they have beneficial functions such as cellular signaling and defense against pathogens. Think of a video game: for each free radical, one antioxidant is needed for balance. When there are more free radicals than antioxidants, this imbalance is known as oxidative stress, damaging cells, tissues, and important molecules such as DNA and proteins.

There is no set adequate amount of antioxidants to be consumed throughout the day, not to mention individuality. But we know that free-radical production has increased. The first suggestion is to seek ways to get rid of the excesses by following Dr. José Roberto's advice in this book and eating colorful and varied foods. Whenever possible, prioritize seasonal organic fruits and vegetables and incorporate seasonings such as turmeric, ginger, cinnamon, cloves, and oregano into your routine.

The easiest way to identify foods rich in antioxidants is by their color. The pigments are compounds with antioxidant action, such as red and purple foods like tomato, red cabbage, beets, strawberries, plums, and blackberries, rich in anthocyanins and lycopene. Orange and yellow foods like tangerines, starfruit, papaya, mango, carrots, and pumpkin, rich in beta-carotene. Green foods like kale, spinach, broccoli, kiwi, and avocado, rich in phenolics and lutein. White foods like garlic, banana, onion, cabbage, and cauliflower, rich in allicin and indoles.

Supplements are important and often essential. But never underestimate the power of basic habits. The simple things that work. Have you noticed how humanity has returned to the past? How the discussion about feet on the grass, looking at the sky, reducing screen time, taking walks, and eating farm food has never been more popular?

I hope I have contributed so that you can make better choices, achieve healthy aging, and high performance, without dependency, until the last day of life. And, as my worthy husband says, Long Live Longevity!

Priscila Parreira Latalisa de Melo

Nutritionist with postgraduate training in clinical, sports, and oncological functional nutrition, and specialization in fertility and pregnancy follow-up.

BIBLIOGRAPHICAL REFERENCES

General Bibliographical References

- ATTIA, Peter; GANDY, Bill. Outlive: The Art a*nd Science of Living Longer and Better. Translated by* Rogério Bettoni. São Paulo: Intrínseca, 2023.
- DAVIS, D. R.; EPP, M. D.; RIORDAN, H. D. Changes in USDA Food Composition Data for 43 Garden Crops, 1950 to 1999. *Journal of the American College of Nutrition*, v. 23, n. 6, p. 669–682, 2004. DOI: https://doi.org/10.1080/07315724.2004.10719409.
- GØTZSCHE, Peter C. Deadly *Medicines and Organized Crime: How the Pharmaceutical Industry Has Corrupted Healthcare.* Translated by Ananyr Porto Fajardo; revised by Daniel Knupp Augusto. Porto Alegre: Bookman; [S.l.]: Radcliffe Publishing, 2016.
- GREENFIELD, Ben. B*oundless: Upgrade Your Brain, Optimize Your Body & Defy Aging*. [S.l.]: Bentoh Publishing, 2020.
- SOUZA, D. L.; SILVA, A. A. *Nutritional Supplementation: Foundations and Practical Applications*. Rio de Janeiro: Guanabara Koogan, 2018.
- WALKER, Matthew. *Why We Sleep: The New Science of Sleep and Dreams*. Translated by Camila Fernandes. São Paulo: Intrínseca, 2018.
- ROBBINS, Tony. *The Energy of Life: Transform Your Physical and Mental Quality of Life with the Vital Energy of Food and*

Movement. Translated by Nivaldo Montingelli Jr. São Paulo: Best-Seller, 2019.

- HOF, Wim. *The Wim Hof Method: Activate the Full Potential of Your Human Body*. Translated by Aline Storto Pereira. São Paulo: HarperCollins Brasil, 2021.
- SINCLAIR, David A.; LAPLANTE, Matthew D. Lifespan: *The New Science of Aging and the Art of Staying Young*. Translated by Alexandre Raposo. São Paulo: Alta Books, 2020.
- LEMBKE, Anna. *Dopamine Nation: Finding Balance in the Age of Indulgence*. Translated by Clóvis Marques. São Paulo: Planeta, 2022.

Scientific References on Circadian Rhythm, Sleep, and Photobiomodulation

- BASS, J.; TAKAHASHI, J. S. Circadian integration of metabolism and energetics. Science, v. 330, n. 6009, p. 1349–1354, 2010.
- BRAINARD, G. C. et al. Action spectrum for melatonin regulation in humans: evidence for a novel circadian photoreceptor. *Journal of Neuroscience*, v. 21, n. 16, p. 6405–6412, 2001.
- CZEISLER, C. A.; GOOLEY, J. J. Sleep and circadian rhythms in humans. *Cold Spring Harbor Symposia on Quantitative Biology*, v. 72, p. 579–597, 2007.
- HAMBLIN, M. R. Shining light on the head: photobiomodulation for brain disorders. BBA Clinical, v. 6, p. 113–124, 2016.
- KHALSA, S. B. S. et al. A phase response curve to single bright light pulses in human subjects. *Journal of Physiology*, v. 549, n. 3, p. 945–952, 2003.
- KLEPEIS, N. E. et al. The National Human Activity Pattern Survey, NHAPS: a resource for assessing exposure to environmental

pollutants. *Journal of Exposure Science & Environmental Epidemiology*, v. 11, n. 3, p. 231–252, 2001.

- KRAUSE, M. et al. Sunscreens: are they beneficial for health? An overview of endocrine disrupting activity. *Molecular and Cellular Endocrinology*, v. 355, n. 2, p. 292–298, 2012.
- SCHLUMPF, M. et al. In vitro and in vivo estrogenicity of UV screens. *Environmental Health Perspectives*, v. 112, n. 3, p. 239–244, 2004.

Complementary References

- ETTEHAD, D.; EMDIN, C. A.; KIRAN, A. et al. Blood pressure lowering for prevention of cardiovascular disease and death: a systematic review and meta-analysis. *The Lancet*, v. 387, p. 957–967, 2016.
- HAMBLIN, M. R. Mechanisms and applications of the anti--inflammatory effects of photobiomodulation. AIMS *Biophysics*, v. 3, n. 3, p. 337–361, 2016.
- LIEVERSE, R. et al. The influence of season on serotonin turnover and depressive symptoms in patients with remitted major depressive disorder. *Journal of Affective Disorders*, v. 133, n. 1–2, p. 232–237, 2011.
- OLSEN, M. H.; ANGELL, S. Y.; ASMA, S. et al. A call to action and a lifecourse strategy to address the global burden of raised blood pressure on current and future generations: the Lancet Commission on hypertension. *The Lancet*, v. 388, p. 2665–2712, Sept. 24, 2016.
- ROSENTHAL, N. E. et al. Seasonal affective disorder: a description of the syndrome and preliminary findings with light therapy. *Archives of General Psychiatry*, v. 41, n. 1, p. 72–80, 1984.

Scientific References on Sleep and Endocrine Health

- CAPPUCCIO, F. P. et al. Sleep duration and all-cause mortality: a systematic review and meta-analysis of prospective studies. *Sleep*, v. 34, n. 5, p. 585–592, 2011.
- PRATHER, A. A. et al. Sleep and antibody response to hepatitis B vaccination. *Sleep*, v. 38, n. 3, p. 391–398, 2015.
- VAN CAUTER, E. et al. The impact of sleep and sleep loss on neuroendocrine and metabolic function. *Hormone Research*, v. 67, suppl. 1, p. 2–9, 2007.
- WALKER, M. Why W*e Sleep: Unlocking the Power of Sleep and Dreams*. New York: Scribner, 2017.

References on Hormones, Lifestyle, and Adaptogens

- CADEGIANI, F. A.; KATER, C. E. Hypogonadism and lifestyle: a meta-analysis. *Current Opinion in Endocrinology*, 2019.
- HUBERMAN, A. *Huberman Lab Podcast*. Episodes on testosterone, sleep, and hormonal modulation, 2022.
- LUBOSHITZKY, R. et al. Disruption of the nocturnal testosterone rhythm by sleep fragmentation. *Journal of Clinical Endocrinology & Metabolism*, v. 86, n. 3, p. 1134–1139, 2001.
- PANOSSIAN, A.; WIKMAN, G. Effects of adaptogens on the central nervous system and the molecular mechanisms associated with their stress-protective activity. *Pharmaceuticals*, v. 3, n. 1, p. 188–224, 2010.

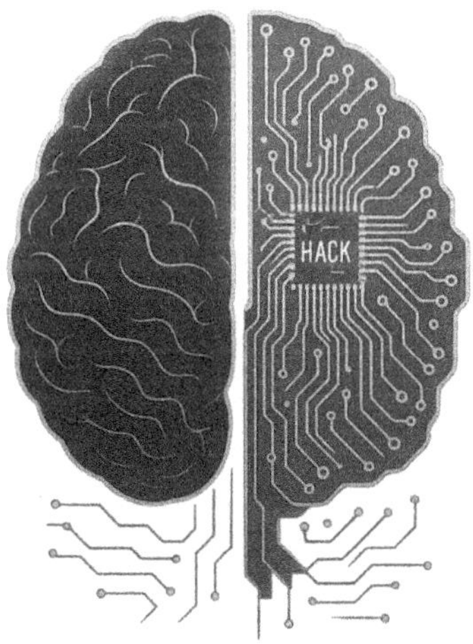
HACK

EDITORA SUARDI

@EDITORASUARDI